1970s
MEMORY LANE

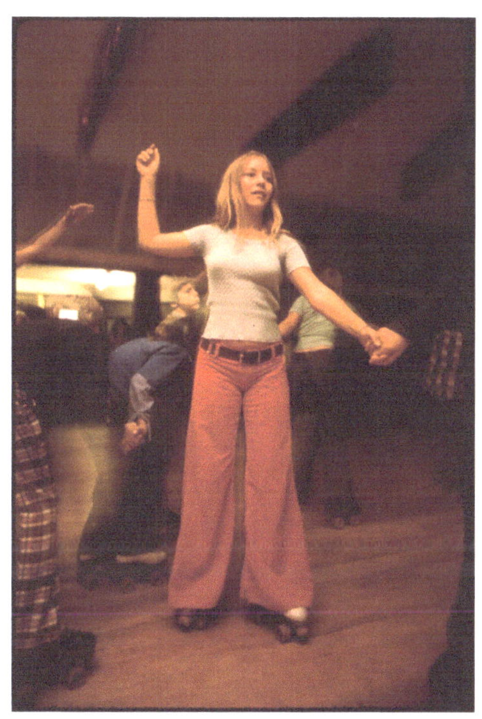

Roller skater, Minnesota, 1976

Compiled by Hugh Morrison

Montpelier Publishing

2021

Cover images:

Front cover (clockwise from left): President Carter. Troops in Vietnam. Philco portable TV. Lynda Carter as Wonder Woman. 'No gas' sign from 1973 oil crisis. Skylab in orbit, 1973.

Rear cover (clockwise from top): Space Shuttle test crew, 1976. Well dressed couple, Chicago, 1975. 1970s 'suitcase' rcord player with autochanger. Darth Vader from the 1977 film *Star Wars*. Singer David Cassidy. President Richard Nixon.

Credits: Chicago Transit Authority, Pal Schiffer, Thrift Store Addict, Sara Luv, Ed and Eddie, Ed Uthman, Joseph Hew, C.Z. Marlin, Dave S, Justso, Public Records Office, Victoria, Erwin Franzen, John White, David Falconer, German Federal Archives, Allan Warren, Ellecid, David Hume Kennerly, Raymond L. Blazewick, Northampton Museum, Seattle at Work, Angeles Chapter History, Dick Row, A&M Records, Rob C. Croes/Anefo, Dada 1960, Ganzkorperfutter, Museum at FIT, Urbain J. Kinet, Walter Landor and Associates, Tamas Urban, University of Liverpool, Washington Area Spark, Archives New Zealand.

ISBN: 9798713370602

Published in Great Britain by Montpelier Publishing.

Printed and distributed by Amazon KDP.

Home in the 1970s

In the 1970s, houses, particularly in the suburbs, got bigger, and there was a reaction to the modernist styles of the 1960s. The 'ranch' style suburban home was very popular. Many such homes featured traditional elements such as stone fireplaces and wood paneling.

The energy crisis meant that commuting became expensive, so some people moved back into restored old city houses which were closer to their workplaces.

Patterns and colors for wallpaper, carpets and drapes became bolder, with geometric and paisley designs. Browns, oranges and greens were common.

Entertaining became less formal, and back yard decking and basement 'dens' became popular. Homes were often built on two levels, known as 'split level'.

Couches and chairs got more comfortable; many such as the 'Lazy Boy' could recline at the pull of a lever.

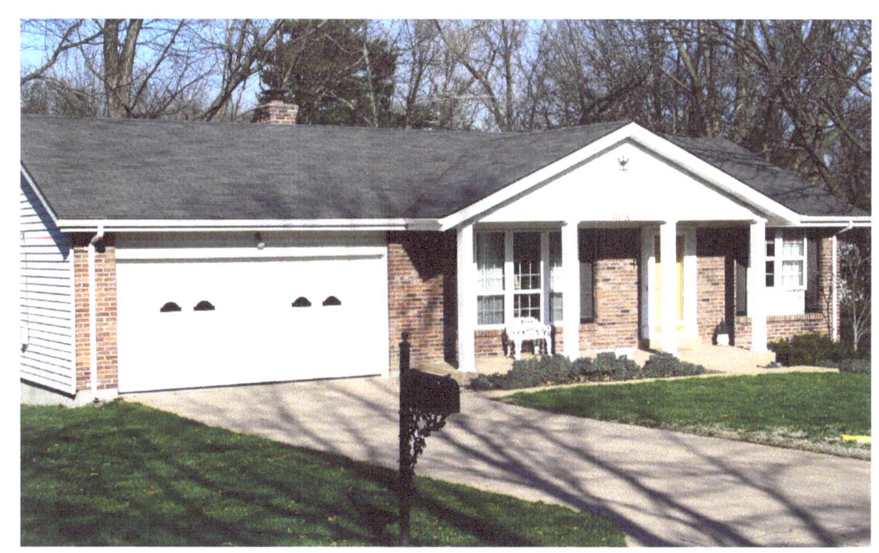

Left: a 1970s ranch house with classical detail and large garage.

Home in the 1970s (continued)

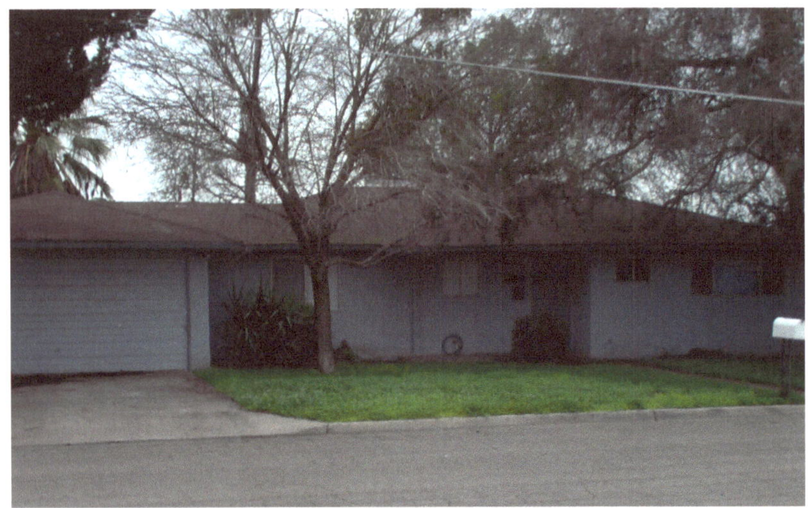

A simple ranch-style house, California.

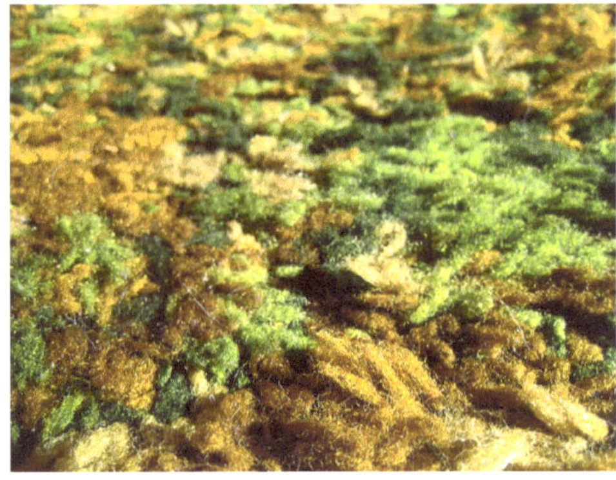

Above: close-up of a 1970s shag-pile carpet design.

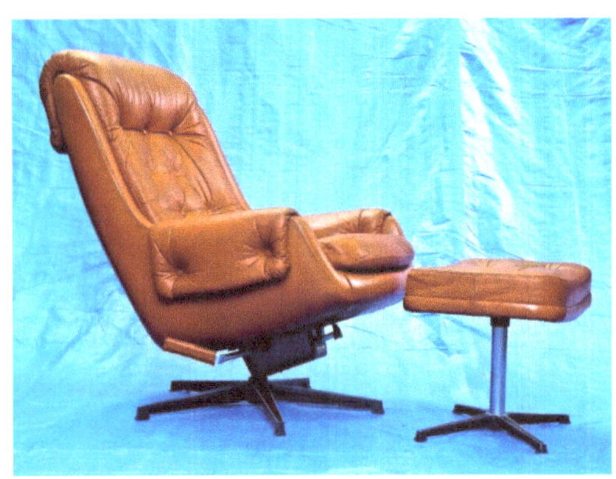

Left: leather lounger with stool.

Right: pendant light.

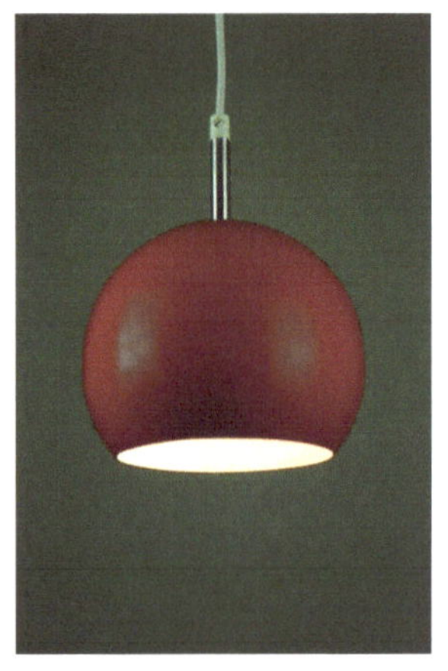

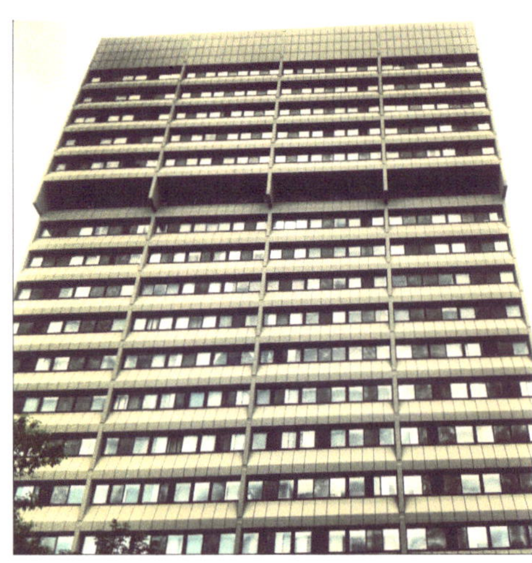

A split-level house.

Apartments, Minneapolis.

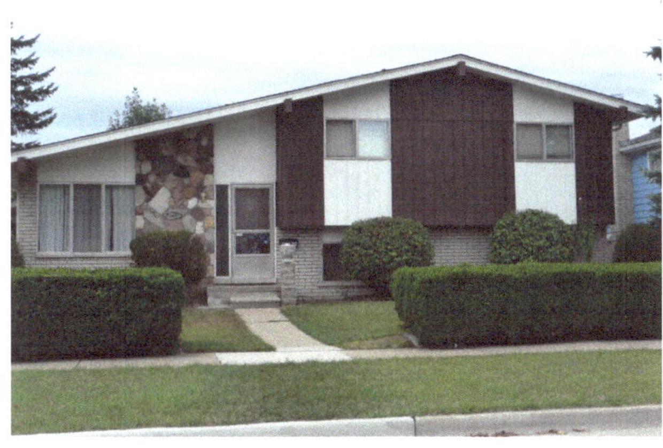

A modern house with stone detail.

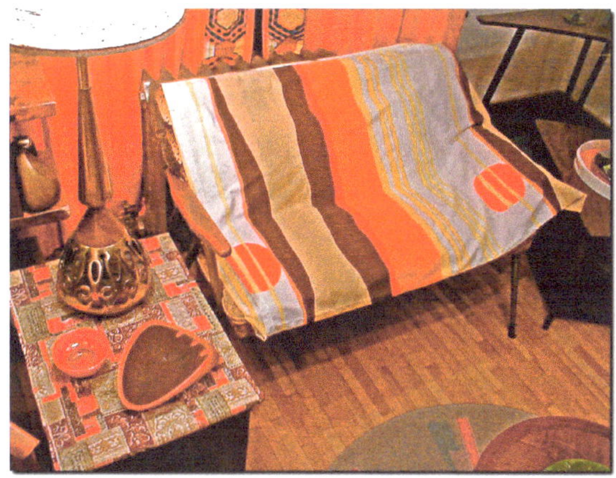

Orange was a popular color for couches and drapes.

Right: interior of an 'A' frame house with timber wall cladding.

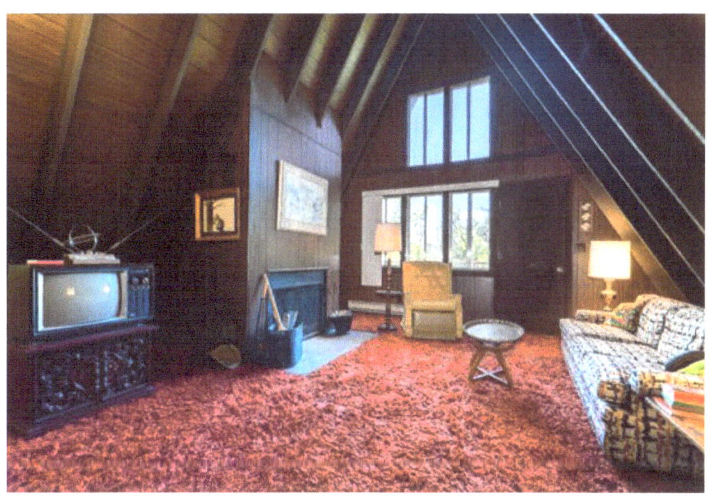

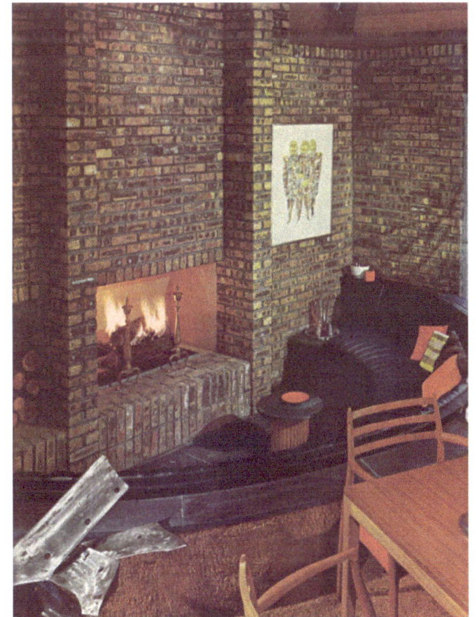

Ranch style fireplace.

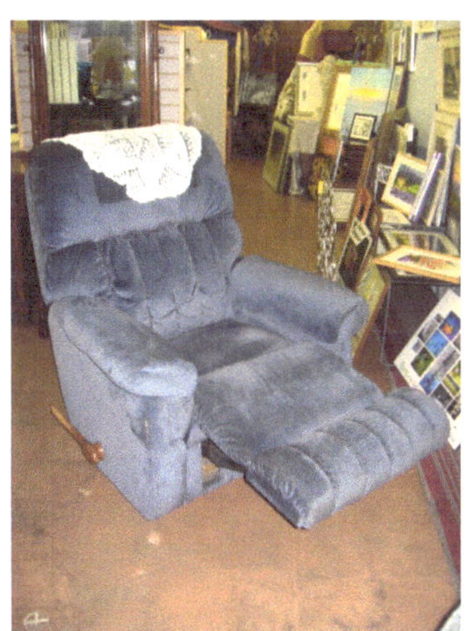

Recliner or 'Lazy Boy' armchair.

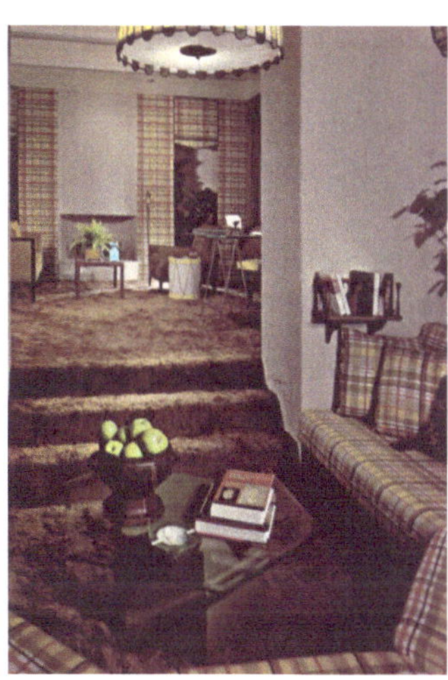

Plaid furnishings.

Travel in the 1970s

In the 1970s, there was an energy crisis, with gasoline shortages and long lines at gas stations. People began to drive smaller cars (compacts and sub-compacts) which needed less gas, such as the Volkswagen Bug and the Ford Pinto. The bigger 'gas guzzler' cars such as large family station wagons gradually reduced in size during the decade.

Bicycle riding also became more popular. Some cities, such as Seattle, introduced bicycle lanes on the roads. In some cities, public transportation was improved with new subway lines to help people get around. Long distance railroad travel continued to decline, and some railroads closed altogether.

Long distance travel by bus, such as the Greyhound lines, was a budget choice for many people. In 1972 Greyhound introduced the Ameripass, which offered 99 days of unlimited travel for $99.

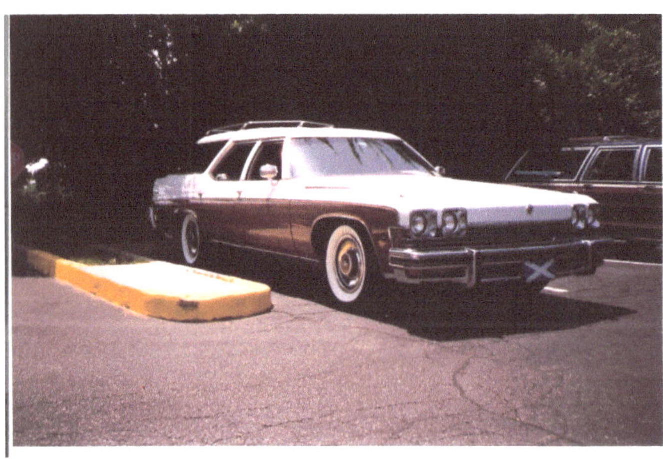

Larger cars such as this Buick station wagon fell out of fashion.

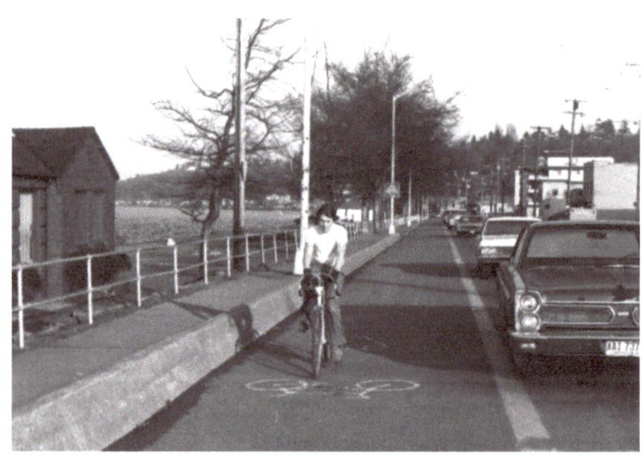

Bike lanes were opened in some cities.

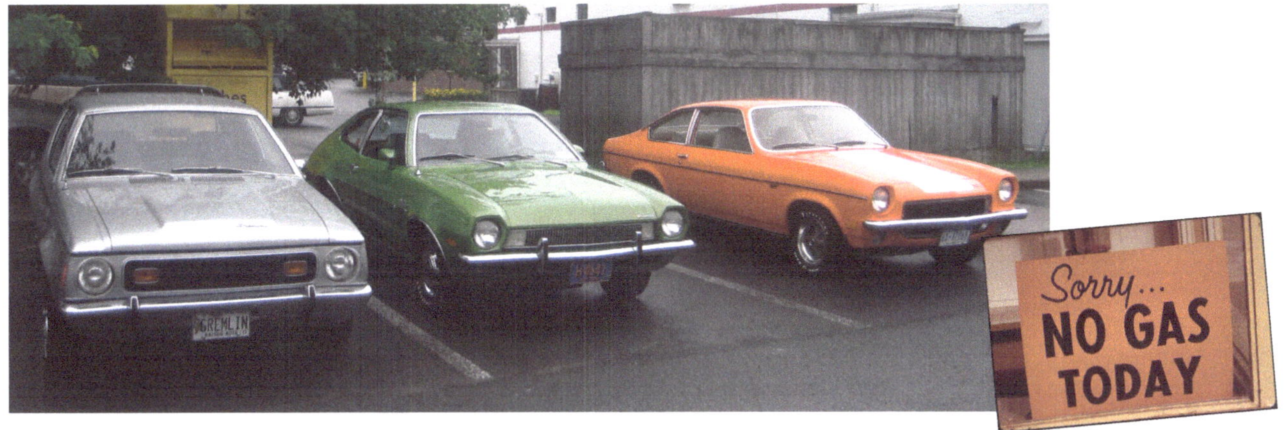

Economical 1970s small cars included (left to right) AMC Gremlin, Ford Pinto, Chevrolet Vega. Inset: 'no gas' sign during the oil crisis.

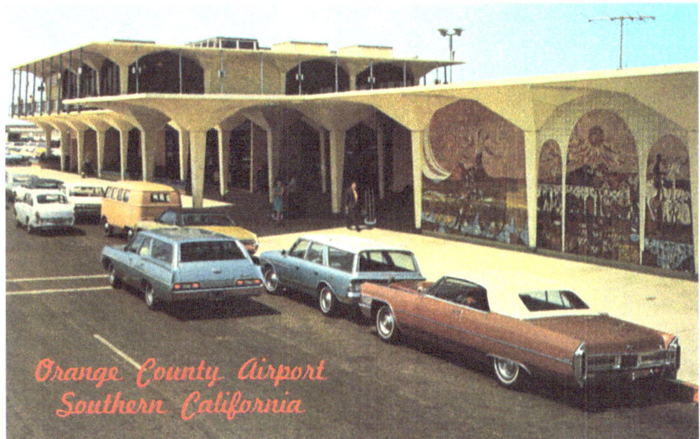

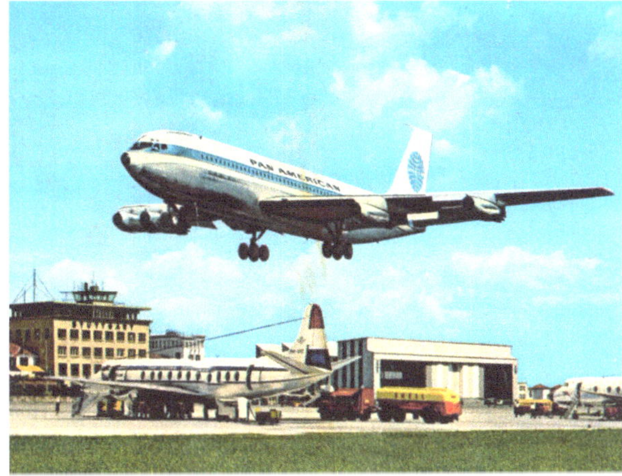

Flying became more common in the 1970s, with new airport terminals (such as the one shown, in Orange County, CA, and new airplanes, such as the Boeing 747 'Jumbo Jet'.

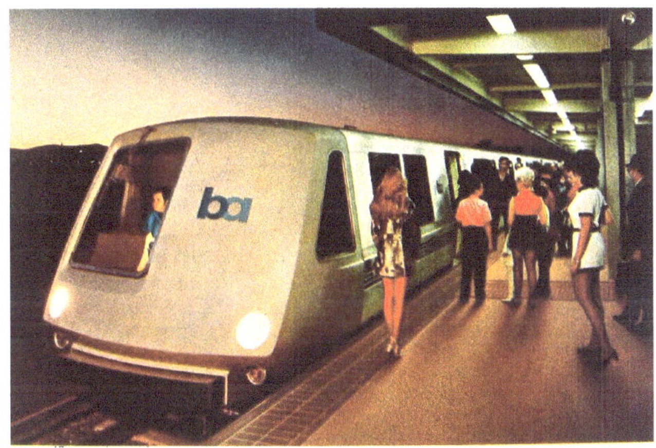

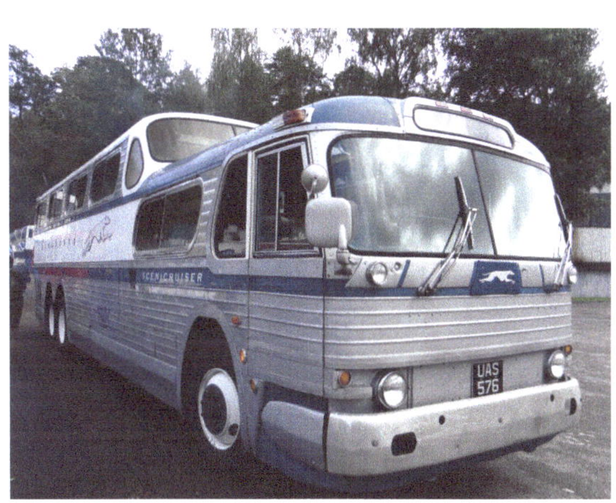

San Francisco's BART subway line.

Greyhound bus.

Work in the 1970s

Big changes happened in American workplaces in the 1970s. Women had always been in the workforce but in the 1970s women in large numbers began to take on jobs in many of the professions, such as medicine, academic and legal work.

Technological changes occurred throughout the decade. In manual jobs, this took the form of improved machinery, automation and safer working practices.

In office jobs, automation and computers also became more common, with fax and telex machines, electric typewriters and computers becoming widespread.

By the end of the decade, small 'microcomputers' that could fit on a desktop were used by many clerical staff.

There was quite a lot of industrial unrest in the 1970s, as many workers went on strike for more pay and better conditions.

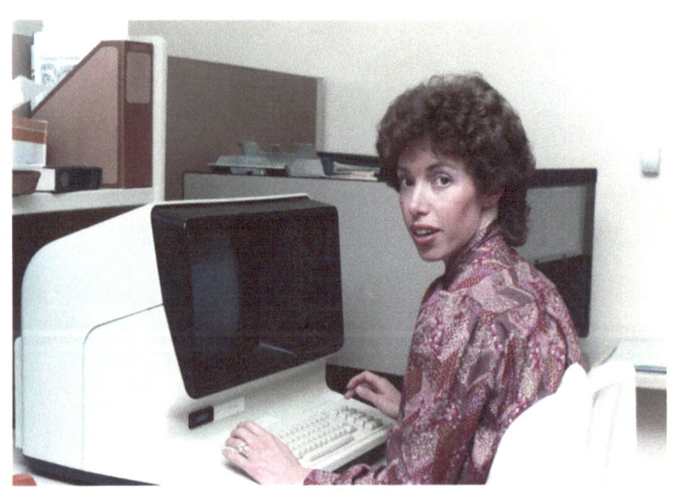

Microcomputer operator, 1979

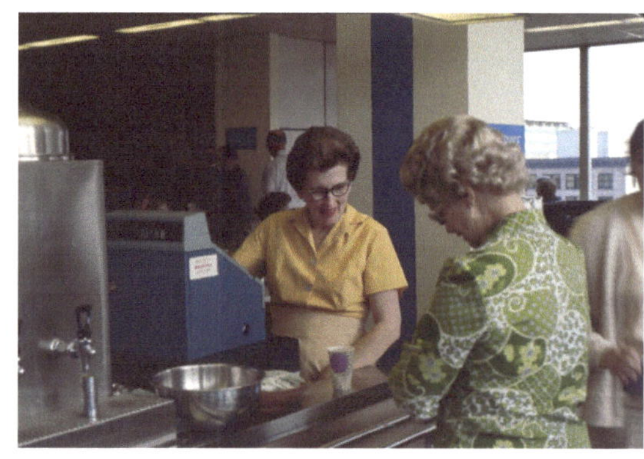

Cafeteria cashier, 1970

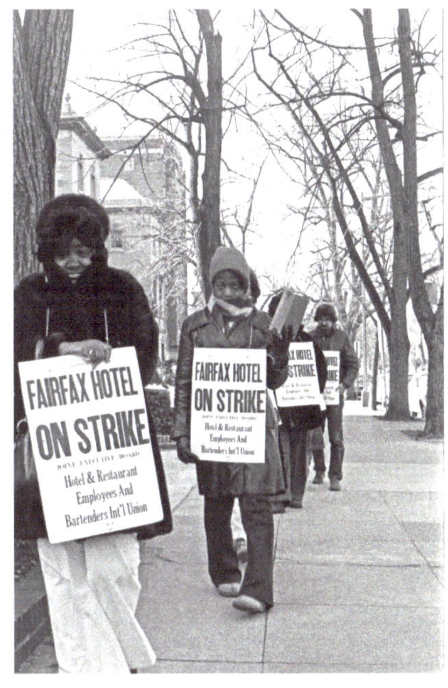
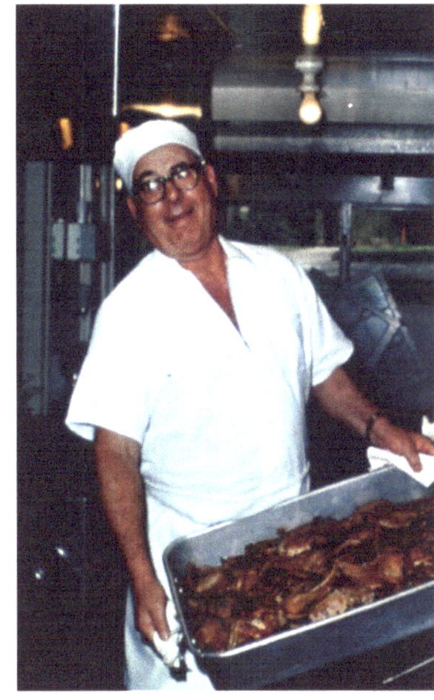

Far left: hotel workers on strike, Washington DC, 1974.

Left: kitchen hand, Seattle, 1977

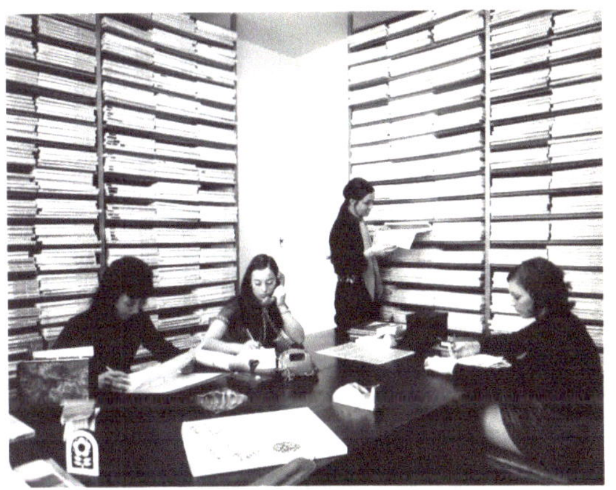

Filing clerks

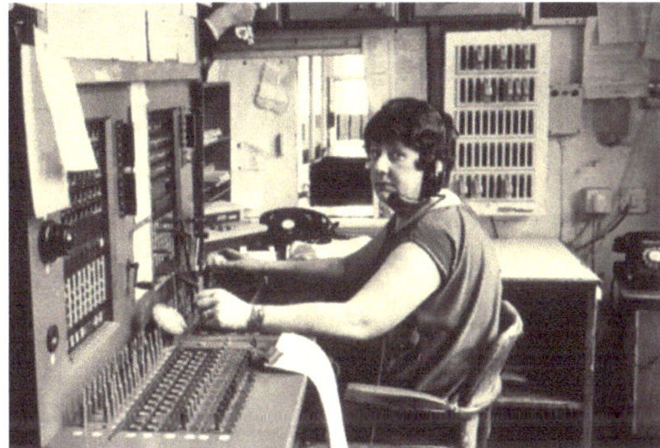

Telephone switchboard operator

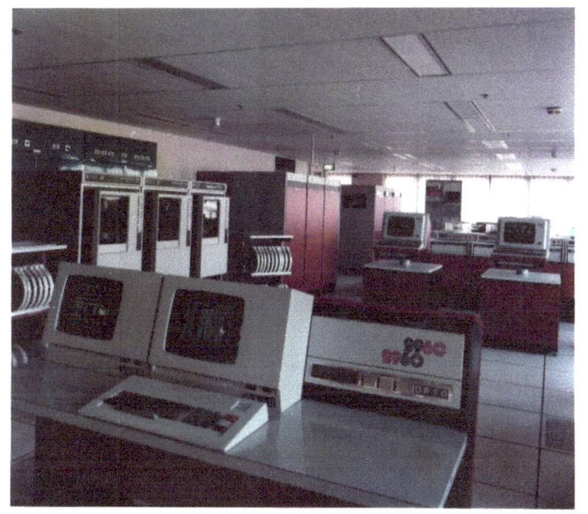

Large office computers

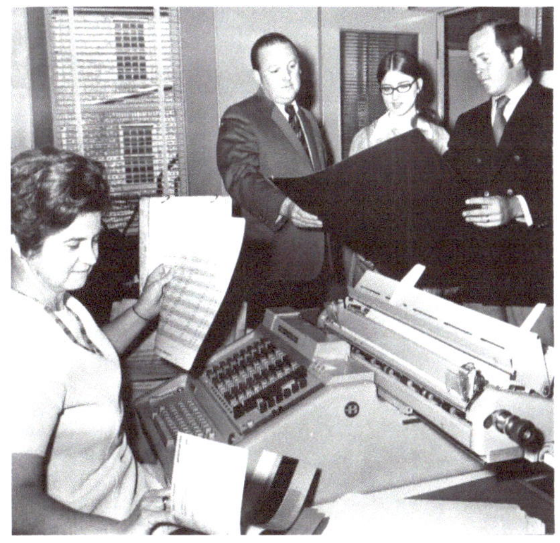

Office workers, 1976.

Leaders in the 1970s

The Presidents and Vice-Presidents of the USA in the 1970s were:

Richard Nixon (Republican) 1969-1974.
Vice-Presidents: Spiro Agnew, Gerald Ford.

Gerald Ford (Republican) 1974-1977.
Vice-President: Nelson Rockefeller.

Jimmy Carter (Democrat) 1977-1981.
Vice-President: Walter Mondale.

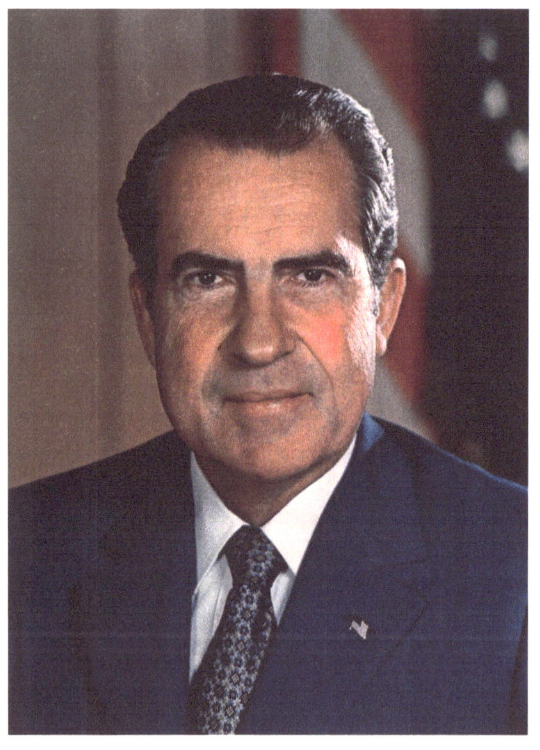

President Richard Nixon (1969-1974).

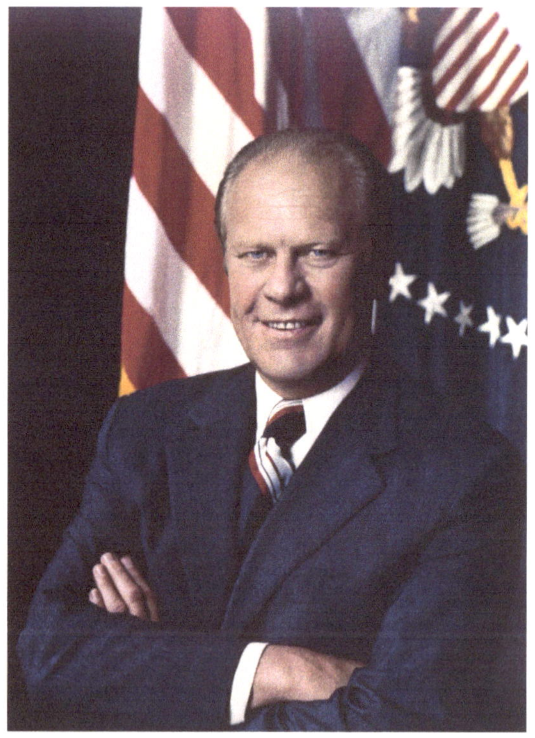

President Gerald Ford (1974-1977).

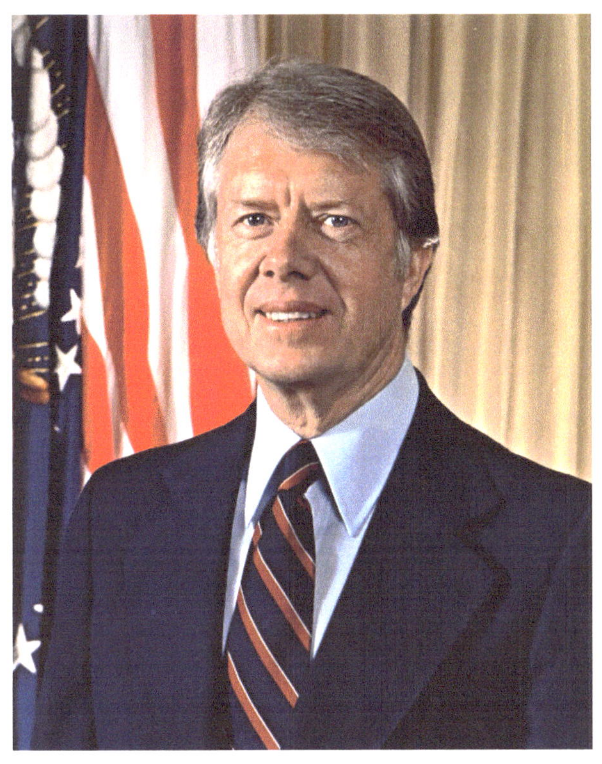

President Jimmy Carter (1977-1981).

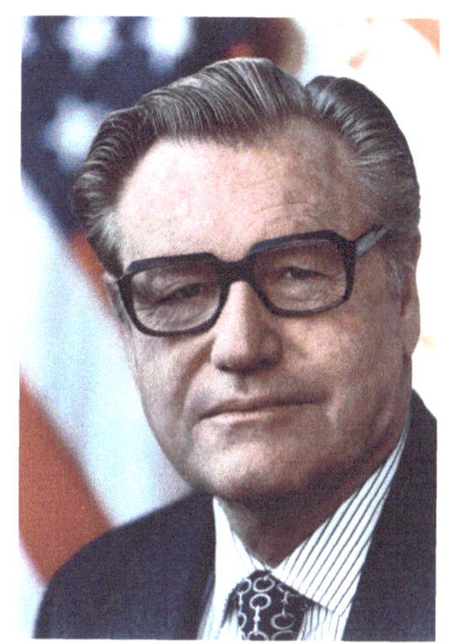

Vice-President Nelson Rockefeller (1974-1977).

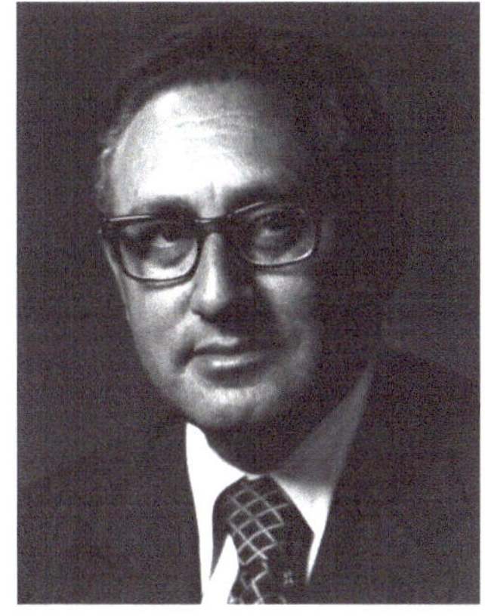

Henry Kissinger, Secretary of State (1973-1977).

Right: Ed Koch, Mayor of New York City (1978-1989).

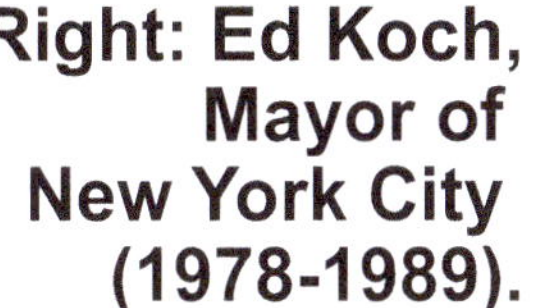

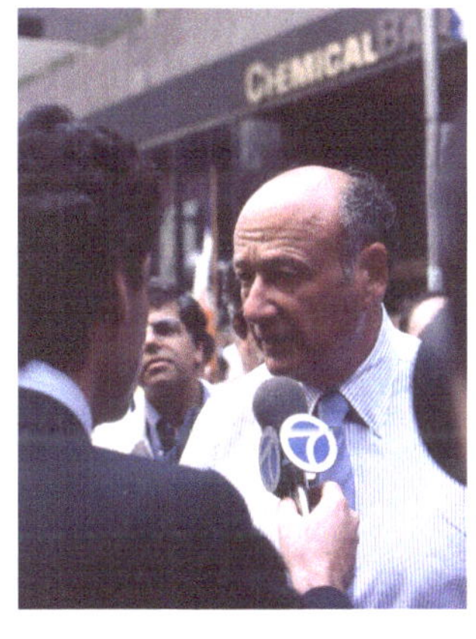

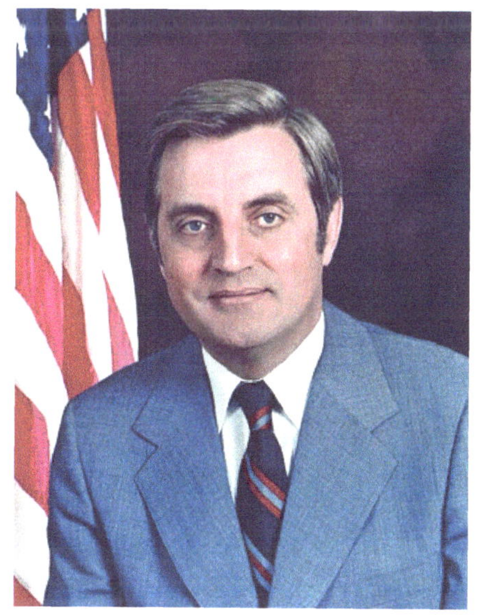

Vice-President Spiro Agnew (1969-1973).

Vice-President Walter Mondale (1977-1981).

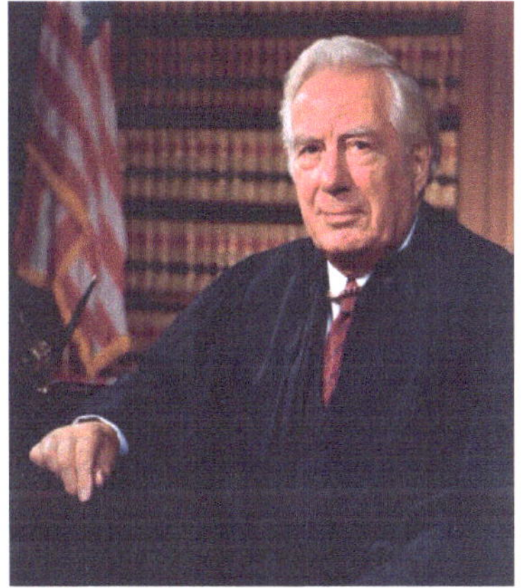

Warren E Burger, Supreme Court Justice (1969-1986).

Music in the 1970s

Two of the biggest events in pop music in the 1970s were the break-up of the Beatles (1971) and the death of Elvis Presley (1977).

Many of the bands and singers from the 1960s continued on the scene, and there were some new arrivals as 'glam rock' became popular. Stars such as Elton John, the Jackson Five and the Osmonds topped the charts.

Disco music was very popular in the later 1970s with bands such as the Bee Gees and ABBA, and stars like John Travolta appearing in disco movies such as *Saturday Night Fever.*

By the end of the decade, 'punk' and 'new wave' music, a lot of it from Britain, began to be popular in the US, particularly amongst youngsters.

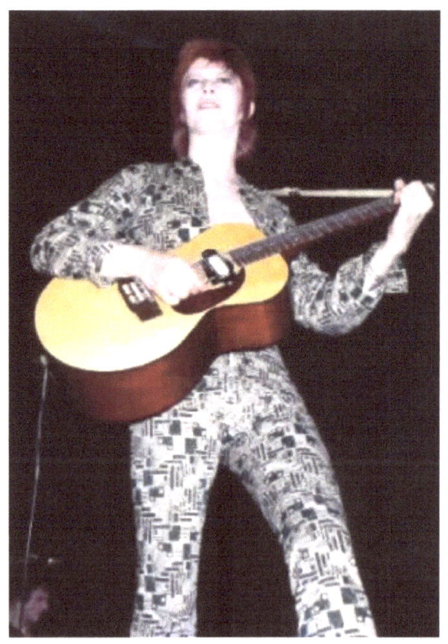

David Bowie.

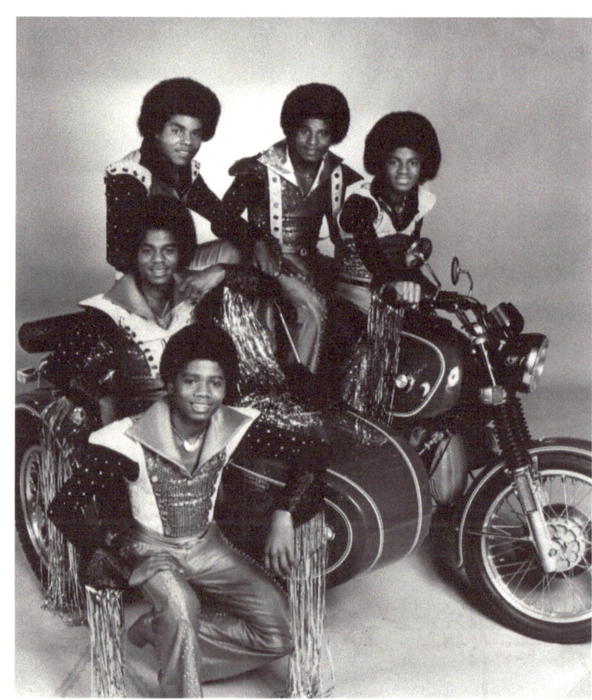

The Jackson Five.

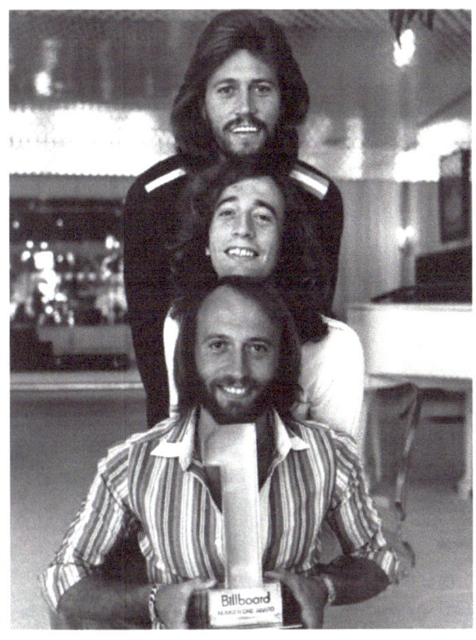

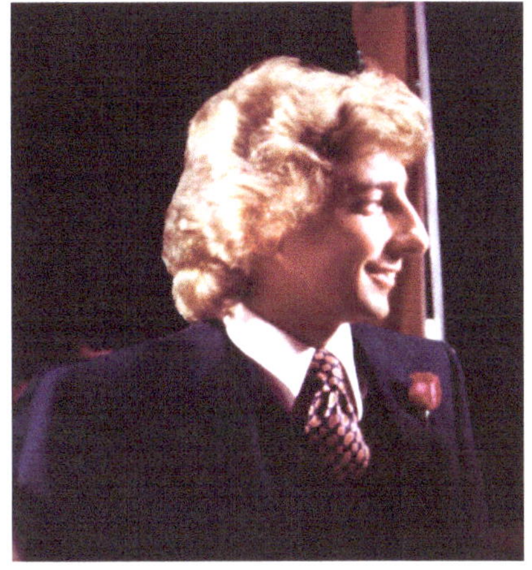

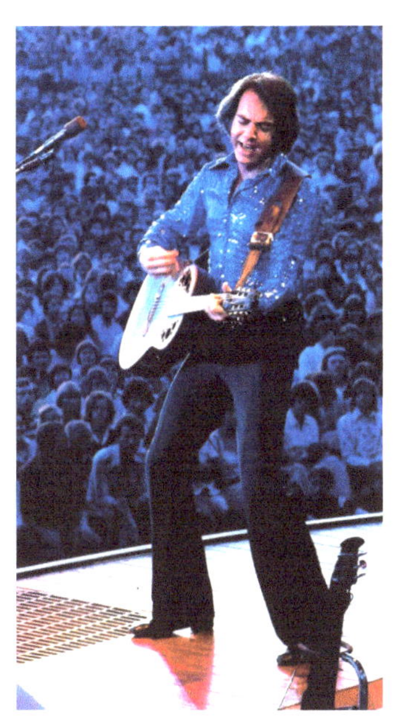

Left: The Bee Gees.
Above: Barry Manilow.
Right: Neil Diamond.

Left: Donny and Marie Osmond.

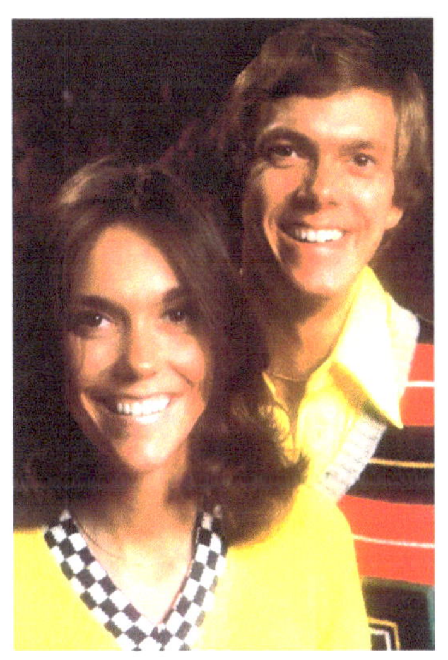

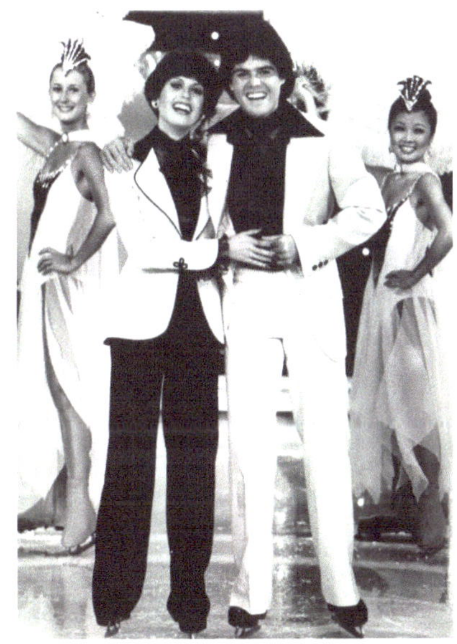

The Carpenters.

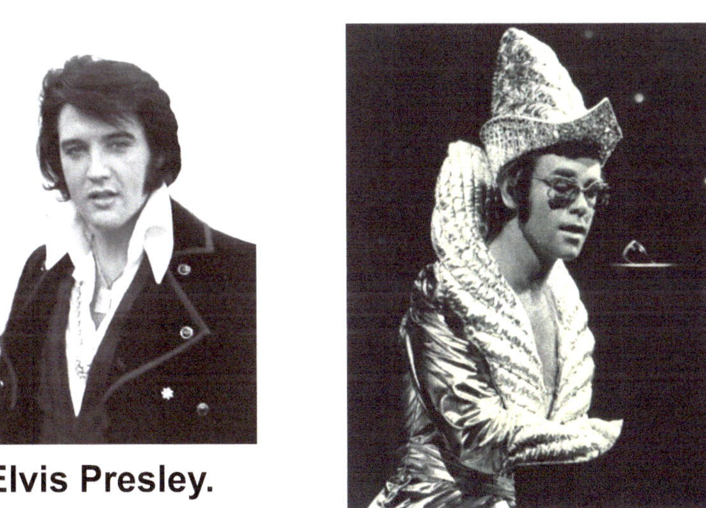

Above: Donna Summer.
Left: Elton John.

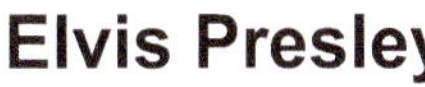

Elvis Presley.

Movies in the 1970s

The numbers of people going to the movies in the 1970s declined for much of the decade, as many people preferred to watch TV.

The movie studios therefore had to tempt back audiences, and they did this by producing a number of 'blockbuster' movies with big budgets and big stars.

Musical movies such as *Grease* and *Saturday Night Fever* made stars out of John Travolta and Olivia Newton John.

Special effects technology improved throughout the decade. Movies such as *The Towering Inferno* and *Jaws* relied on expensive special effects to thrill the audience.

This culminated in *Star Wars* in 1978, which is still one of the highest grossing movies on record.

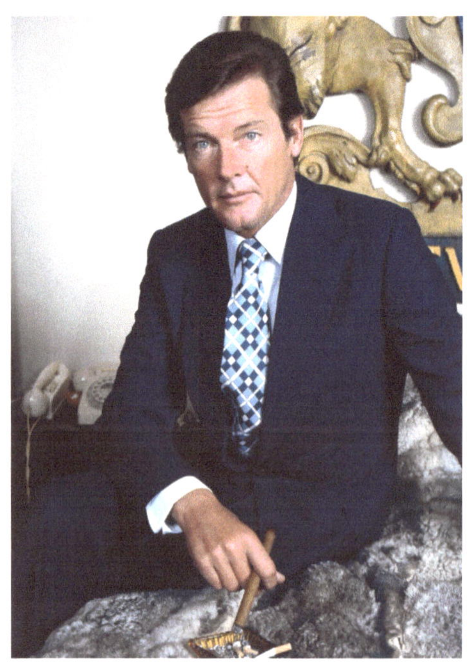

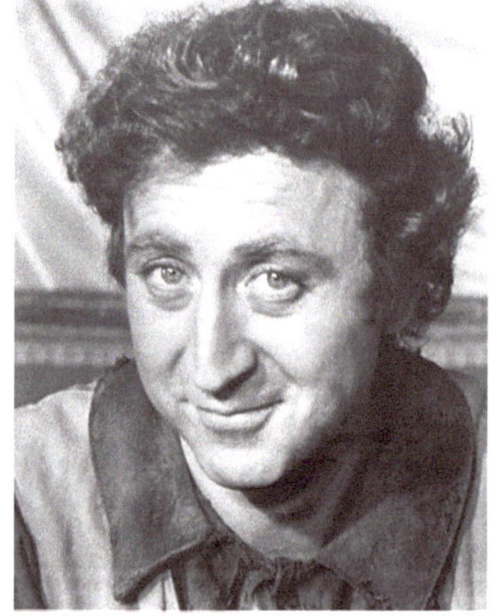

Left: Roger Moore starred as agent James Bond 007.

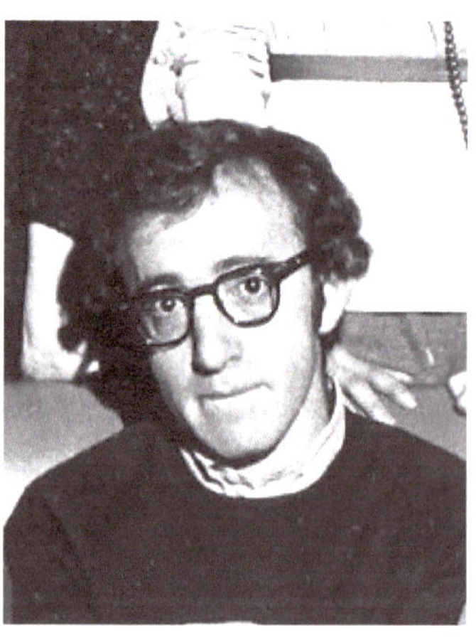

Gene Wilder (above left) and Woody Allen (right) were major comedy stars.

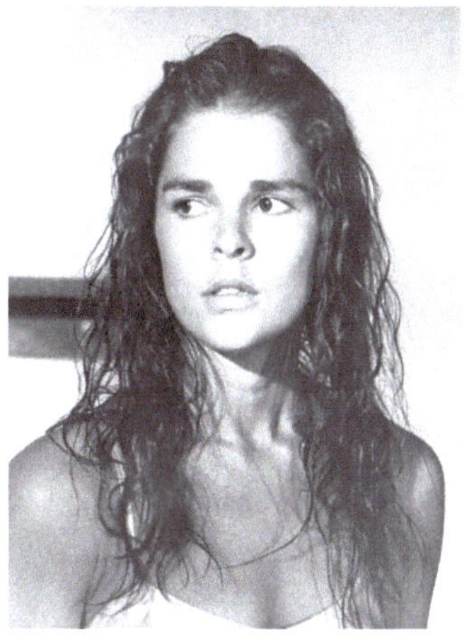
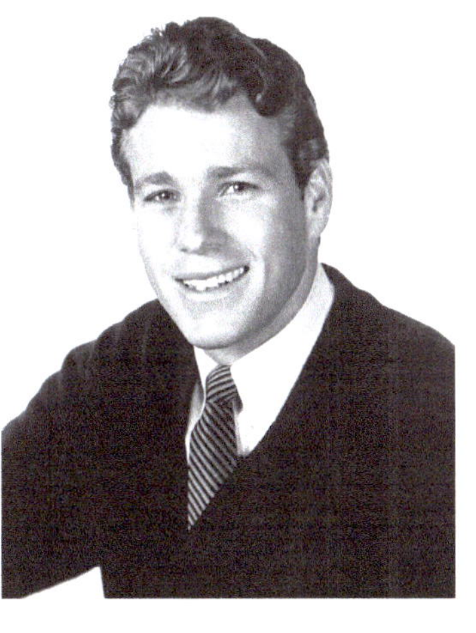

Ali McGraw and Ryan O'Neal starred in *Love Story* (1970).

Olivia Newton-John and John Travolta starred in *Grease* (1978).

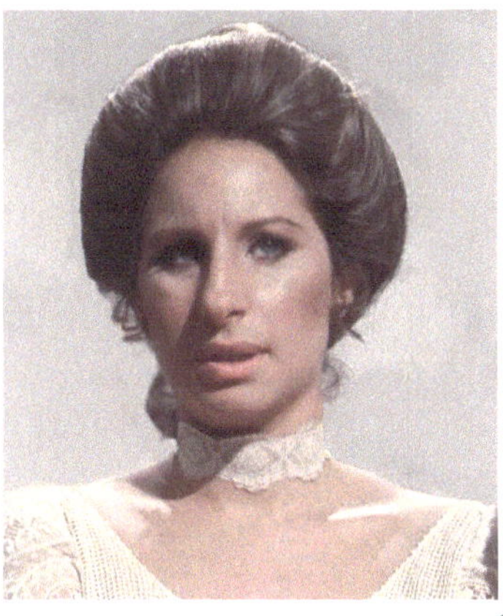

Barbra Streisand starred in *The Way We Were* (1973).

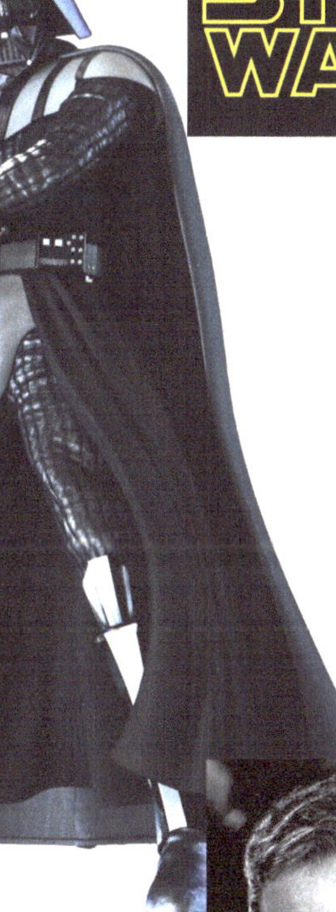

Darth Vader (left) was the villain in *Star Wars* (1978).

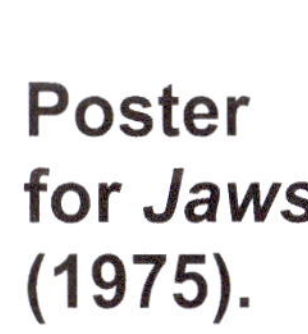

Poster for *Jaws* (1975).

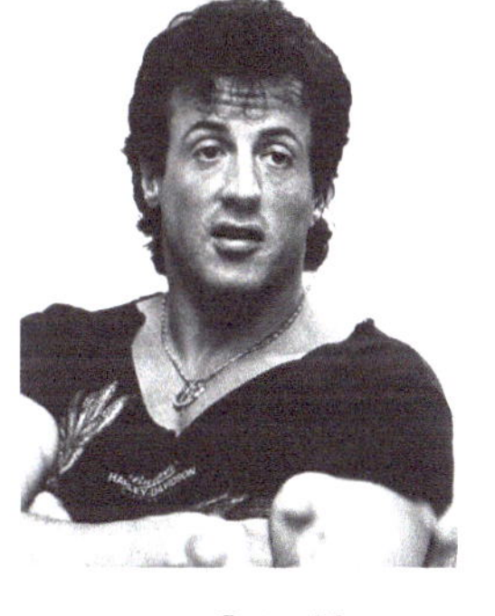

Sylvester Stallone starred in Rocky (1976).

Peter Sellers starred in the *Pink Panther* movies.

Sport in the 1970s

Major league baseball was boosted by color TV coverage in the 1970s. TV's *Monday Night Baseball* coverage was very popular; fixtures increased in the 1970s from 154 games to 162 per year.

In football, the NFL and AFL merged in 1970, and TV's *Monday Night Football* launched the same year; the NFL Super Bowl also became one of the nation's most watched programs.

The Olympic Games were held twice in the 1970s; in Munich, West Germany (1972) and Montreal, Canada (1976).

In the 1970s, fitness became fashionable, which resulted in some new sports becoming popular. Skateboarding, table tennis, marathon running and jogging all gained huge numbers of followers.

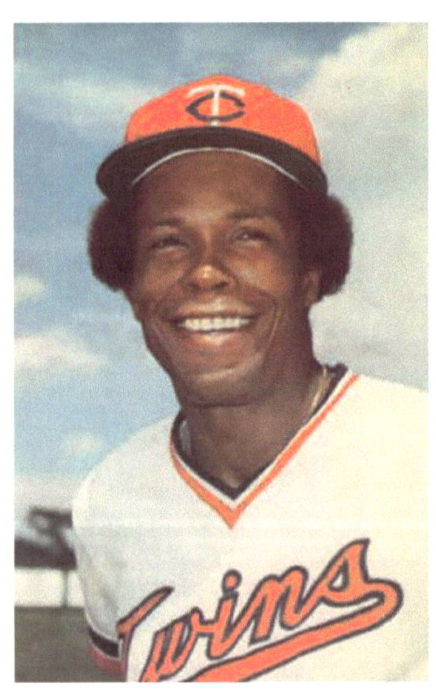

Baseball star Rod Carew.

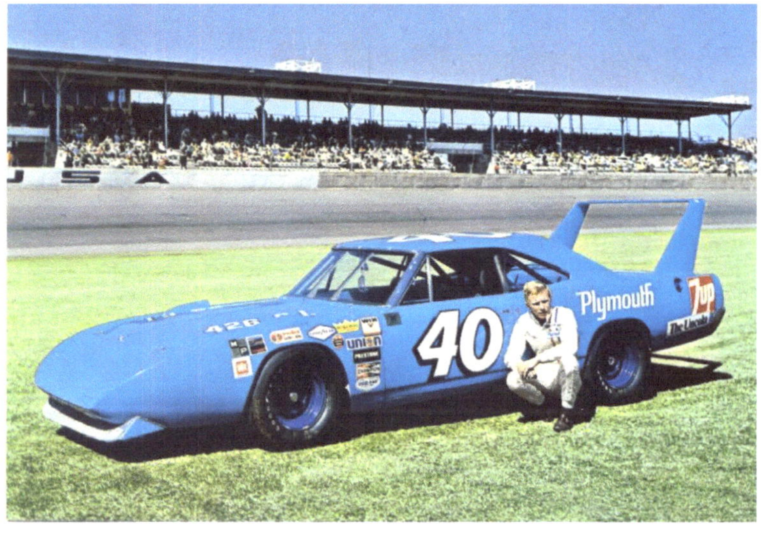

NASCAR driver Pete Hamilton.

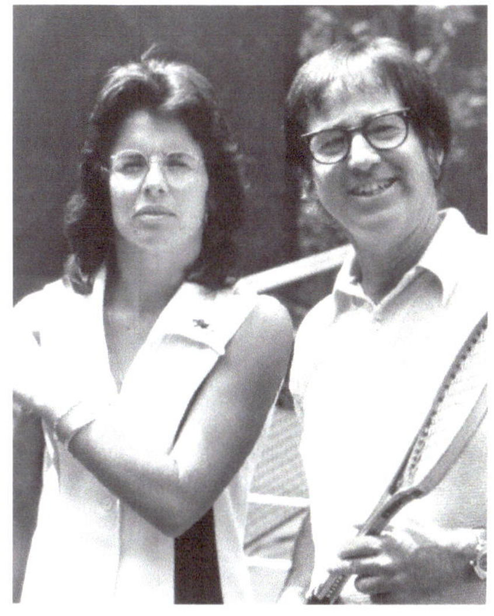

Tennis stars Billie Jean King and Bobby Rigg.

Below: Olympic skier Martha Rockwell.

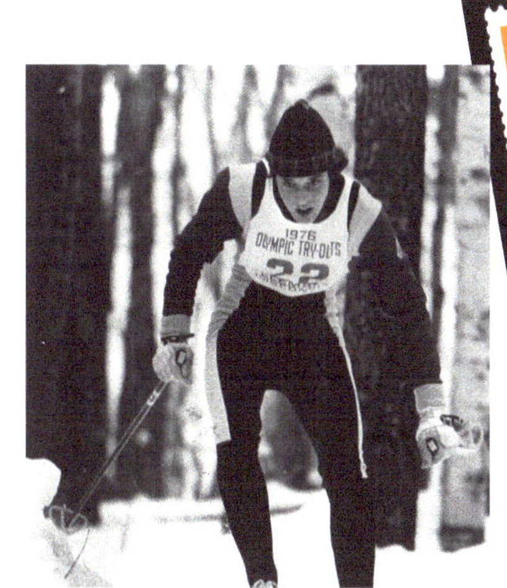

Right: 1972 Munich Olympics stamps.

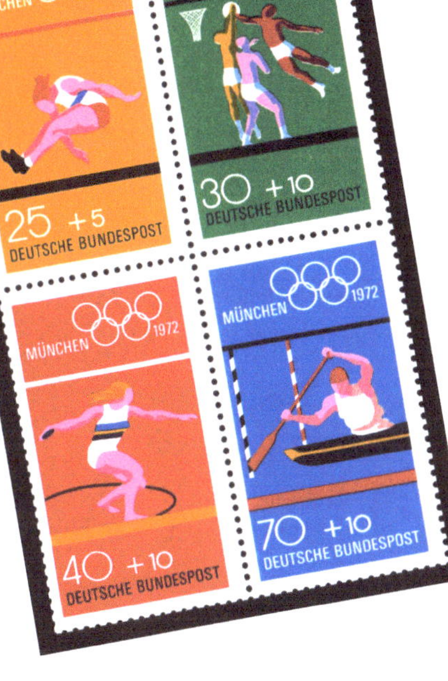

Right: Tennis champ Jimmy Connors.

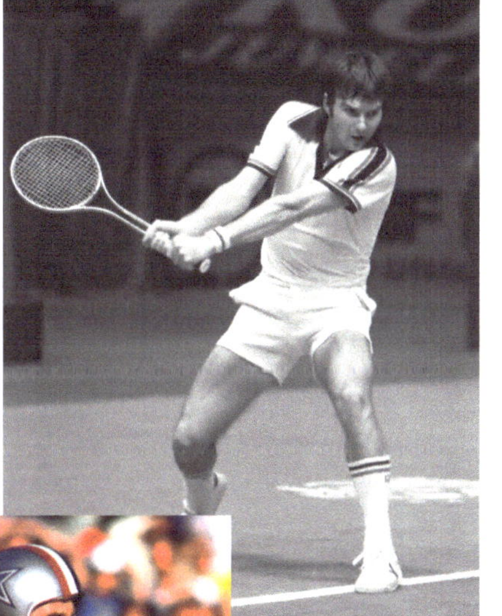

Left: baseball champ Tom Seaver. Below: Connie Hawkins of the Harlem Globetrotters.

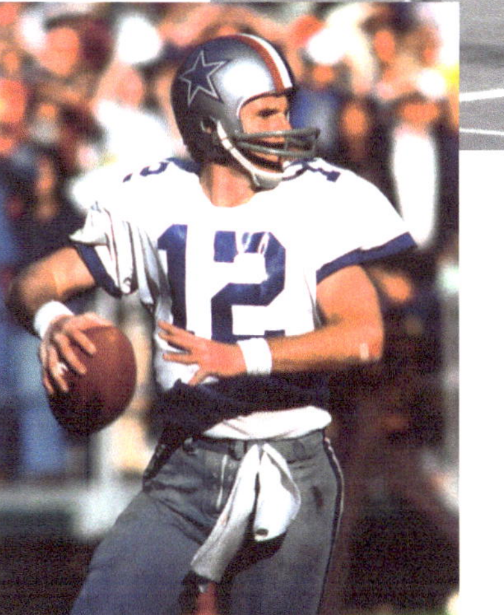

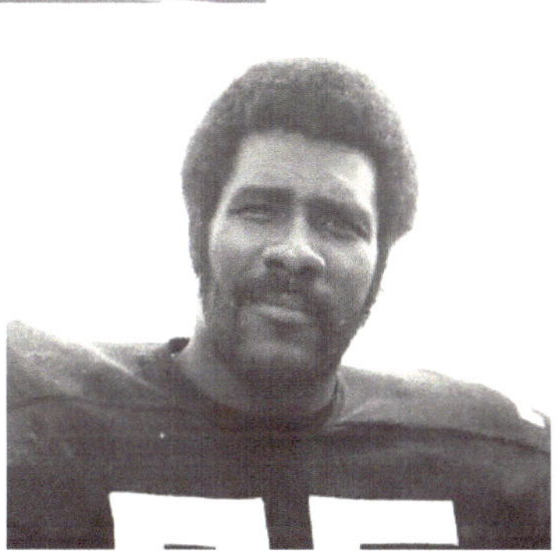

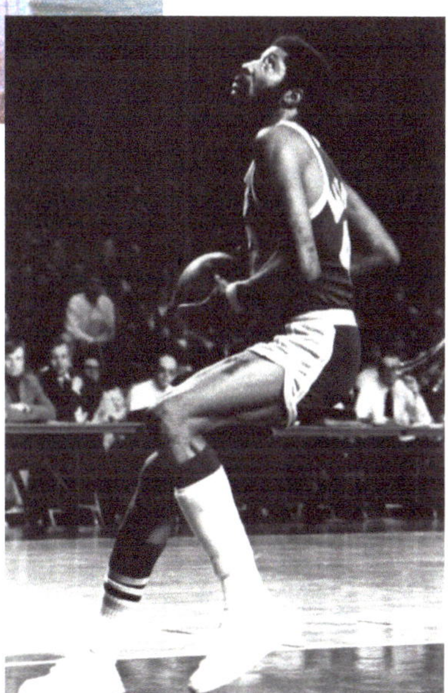

Football champs Roger Staubach (above left) and 'Mean' Joe Green (above right).

TV in the 1970s

TV shows in the 1970s had bigger budgets than in previous decades, which meant that production values were high and stars became very well paid.

TV sports coverage expanded in the 1970s, with Monday Night Baseball, Monday Night Football and the NFL Super Bowl first broadcast in this decade.

TV drama began to explore new themes such as racial equality and women's liberation, which had not been covered much in earlier shows.

News coverage underwent big changes, with more reports on location. The Vietnam War was the first to be televised, and anchormen such as Walter Kronkite reported from the front lines.

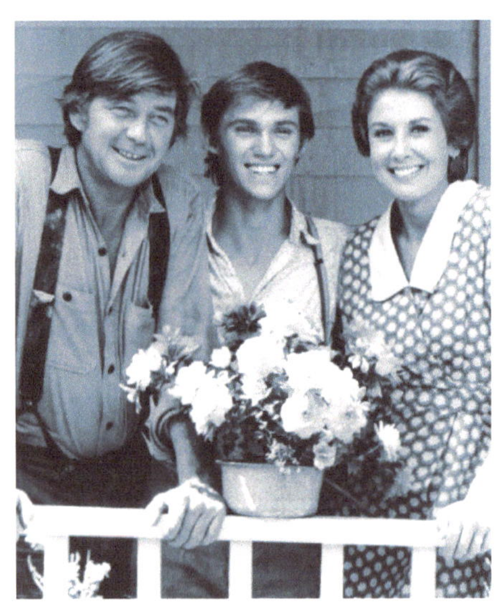

The Waltons.

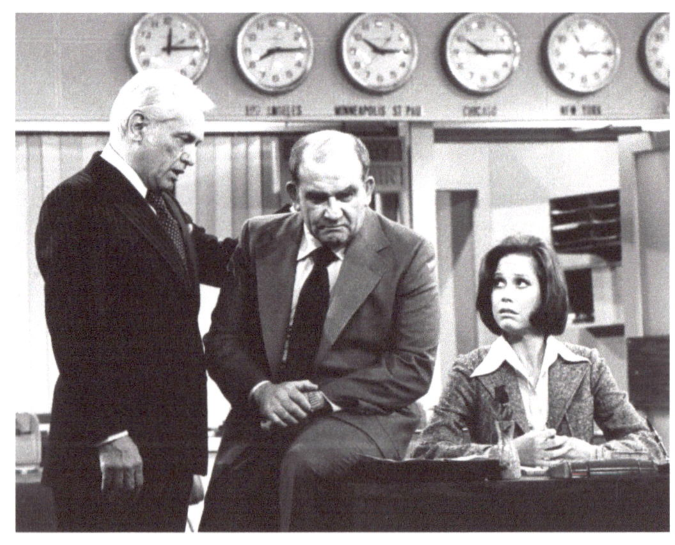

The Mary Tyler Moore Show.

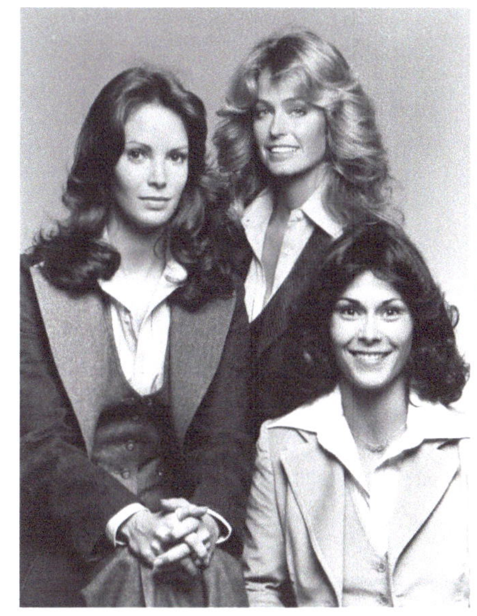

Left: *Charlie's Angels*
Right: *the Rockford Files.*

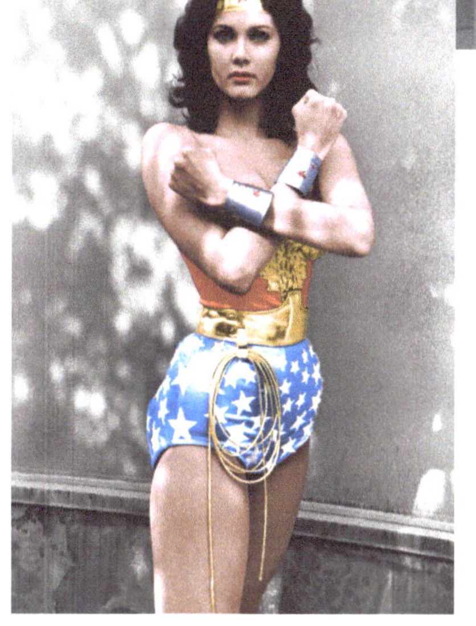

Left: *The Partridge Family.*
Above: *Wonder Woman.*

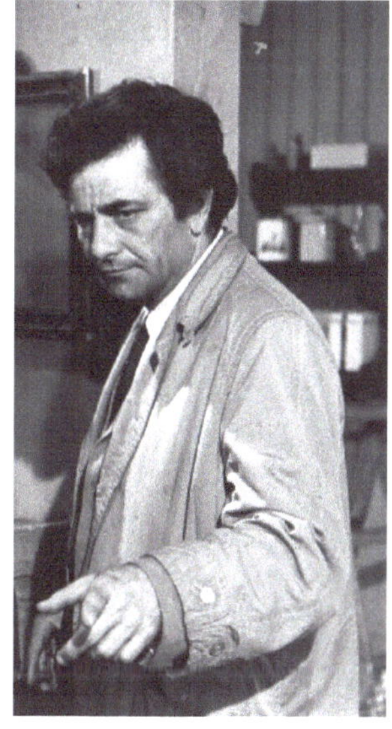

Above: *Columbo.*
Below: Kermit in *The Muppet Show.*

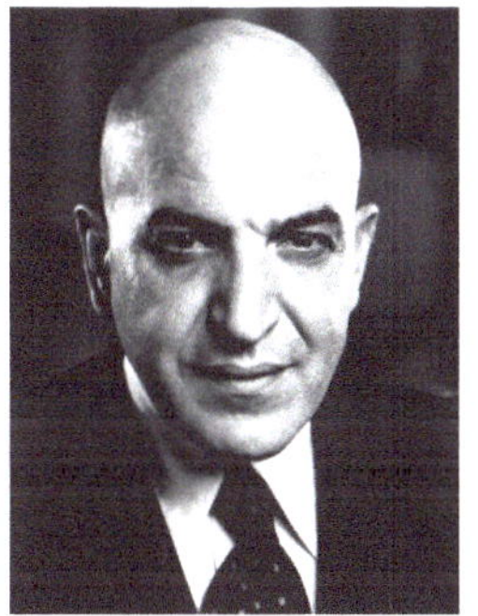

Telly Savalas as *Kojak.*

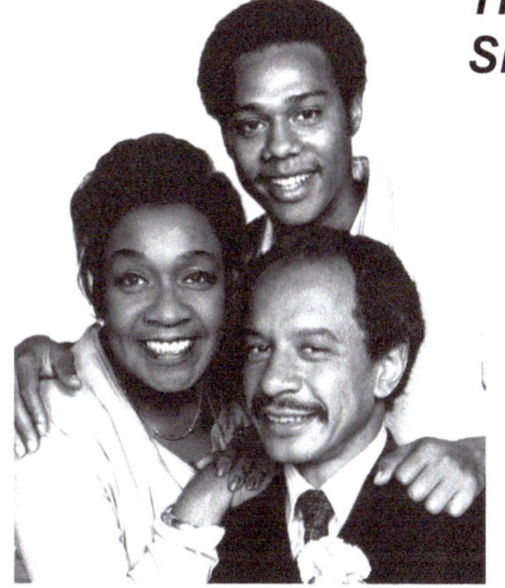

Above: *The Jeffersons.*
Left: Walter Kronkite in Vietnam.

Vacations in the 1970s

Overseas vacations were originally only for the wealthy. In the 1970s however, that began to change as airplanes got bigger, leading to lower costs. It became possible to fly to Europe for around $200.

Finally in 1978 the Federal government allowed airlines to set their own prices which led to even lower fares.

The expansion of airlines also meant that there was more choice for those who wanted a domestic vacation. Resorts such as Disneyworld opened and there was big growth in areas such as Las Vegas.

For those who went on vacation with their cars, there were a lot more motels to chose from. Chains such as Motel 6 expanded during the 1970s, making it possible to stay in comfortable rooms at reasonable prices.

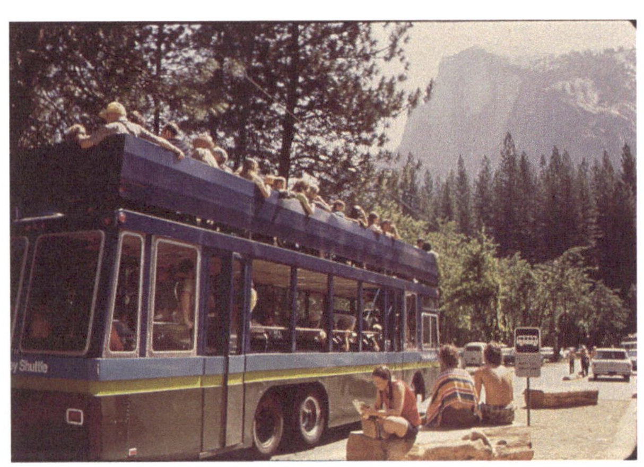

Tour bus at Mammoth Mountain, California, 1975.

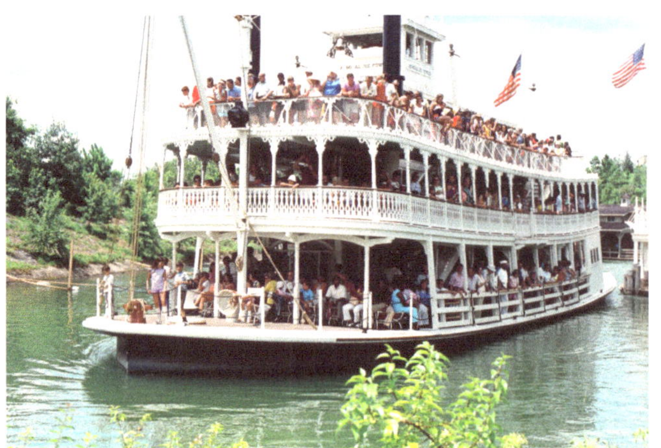

Steamboat ride, Disneyworld, Florida, 1972.

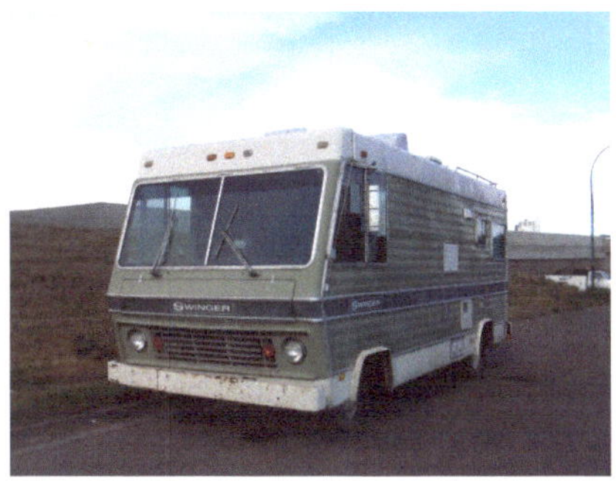

Left: Vacations in RVs became very popular in the 1970s.

Below: luxury motels became more common.

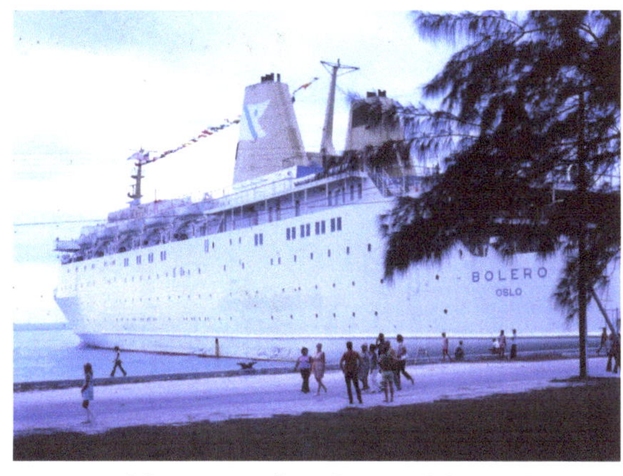

Above: Cruise ship, Key West, Florida, 1973.

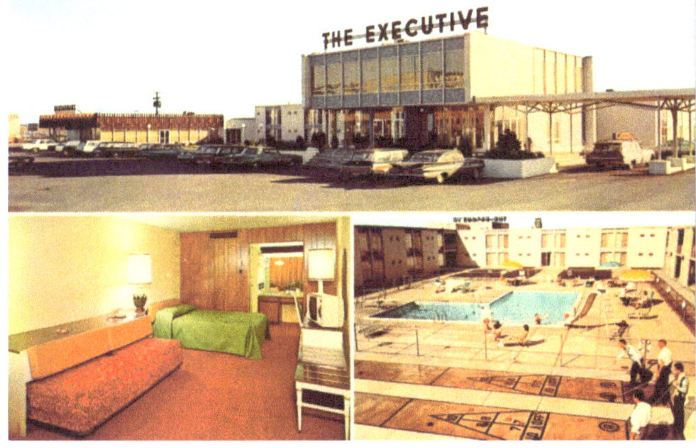

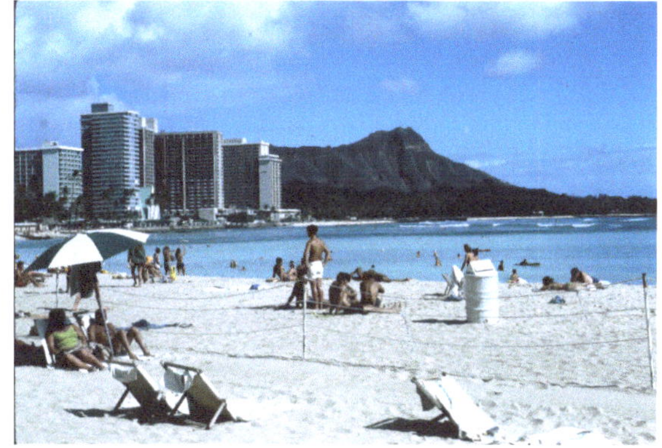

Above and below: Hawaii became a popular vacation destination in the 70s.

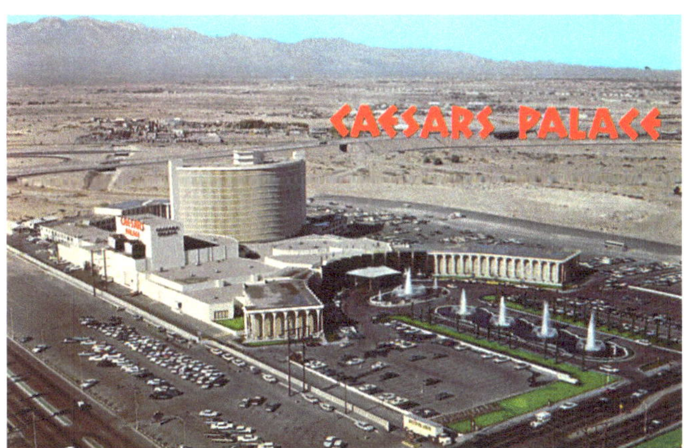

Above: the resort of Las Vegas grew rapidly in the 70s.

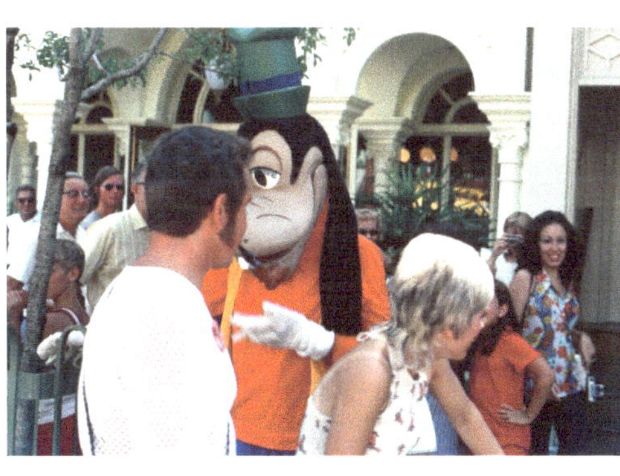

Right: vacationers meet Goofy at Disneyworld, Florida, 1972.

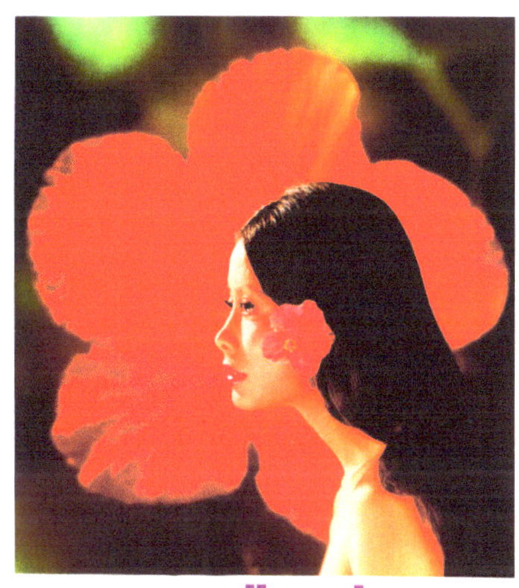

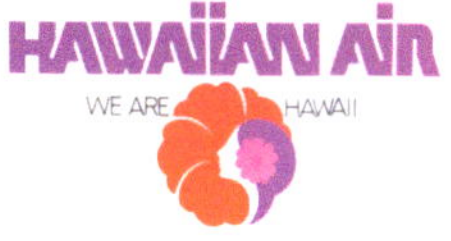

Fashion in the 1970s

Womens' fashion in the early 1970s largely followed that of the 1960s, with bright colors and 'psychedelic' patterns. One big change was the fashion of the ankle length 'maxiskirt', in stark contrast to the miniskirts of the previous decade.

As the 70s progressed, styles became more conservative; although by the late 1970s, sportswear such as jogging suits and sweat pants began to be seen. Styles for young men continued to become more casual, and long hair and beards became acceptable in all but the most conservative circles.

One defining feature of the decade was the popularity of 'unisex' clothing which could be worn either by men or women, such as jeans and denim jackets. Bell bottomed trousers became standard for both men and women.

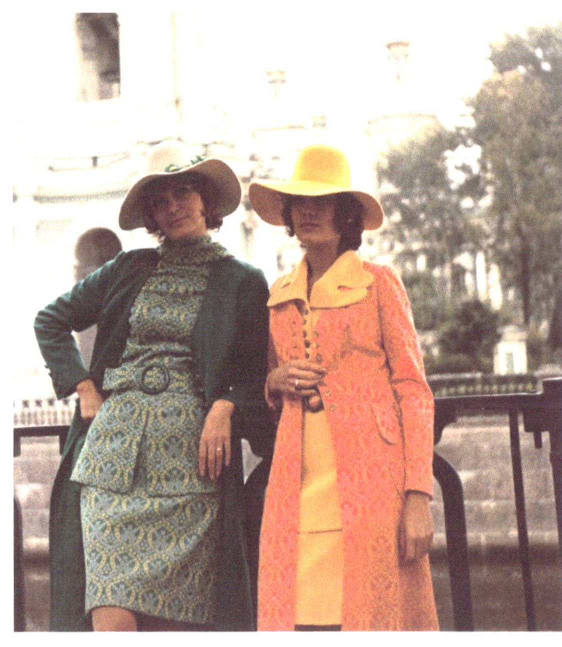

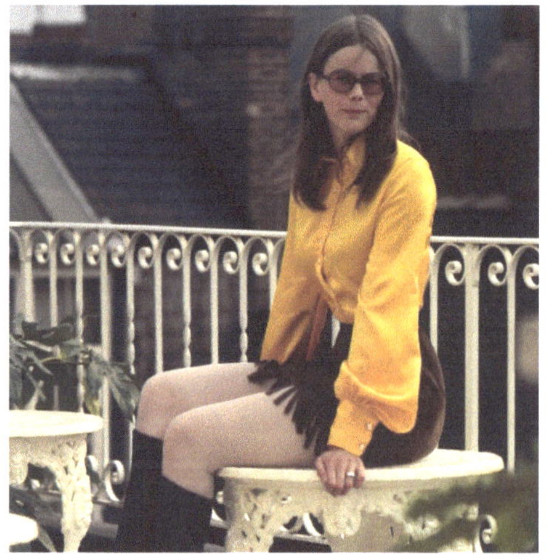

Left: summer coats with co-ordinating hats, 1973. Above: suede miniskirt and boots, 1971.

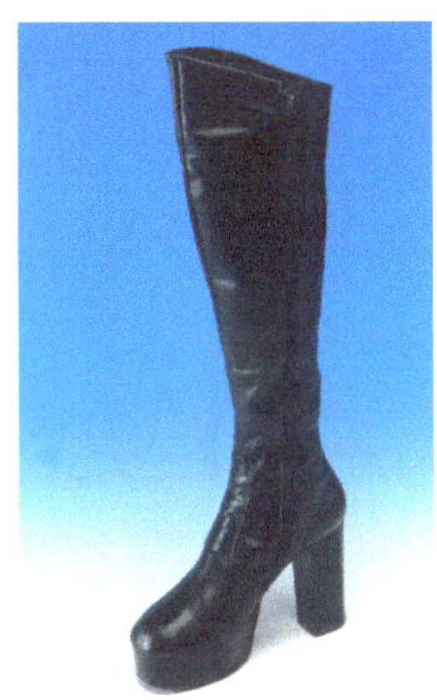

Left: platform boot.
Right: two hair styles of the 1970s: the Afro and the Farah Fawcett Flick.

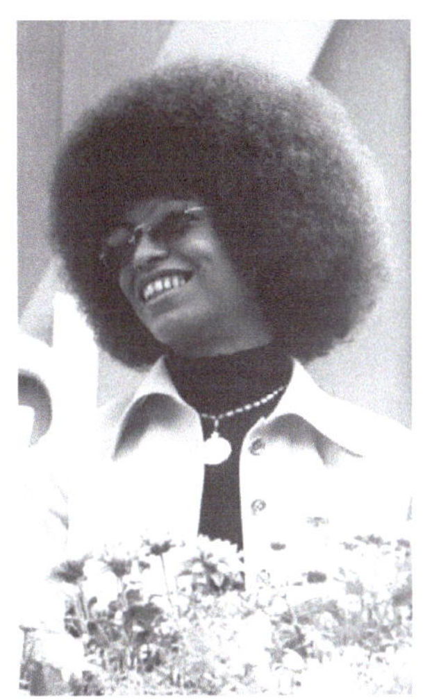

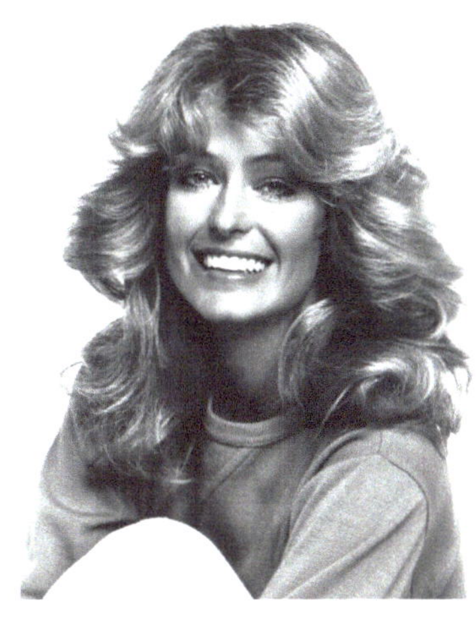

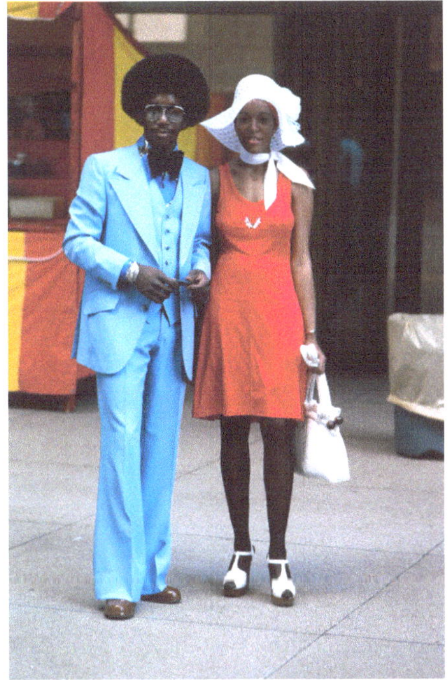

Well dressed couple, NYC, 1975.

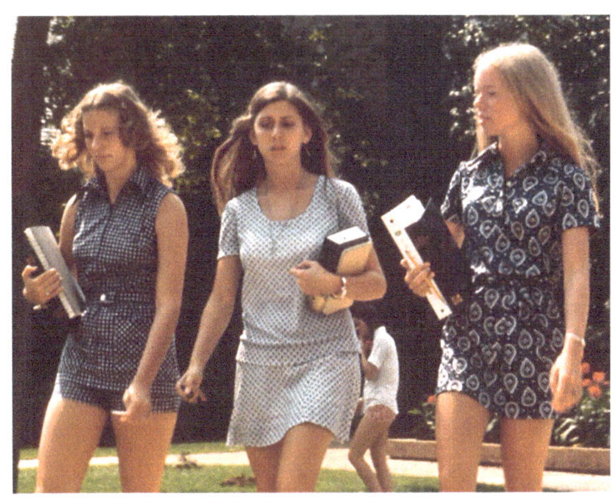

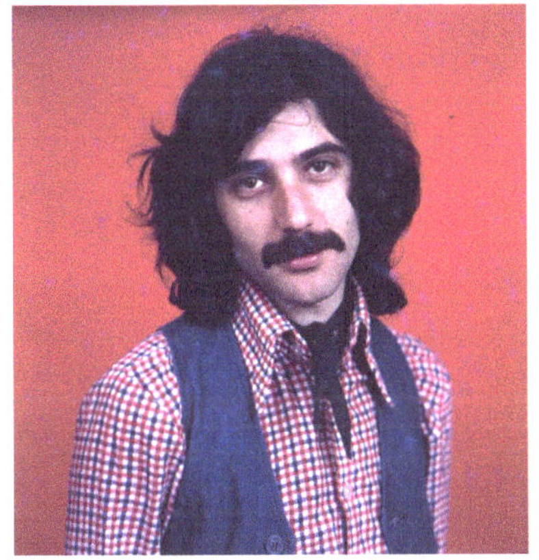

Man with long hair and moustache, 1979.

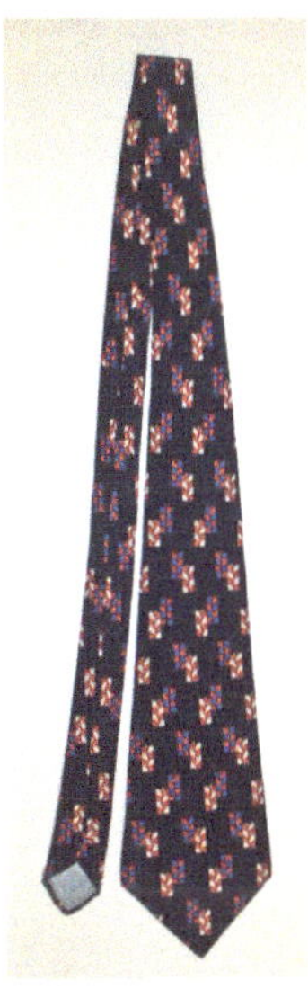

'Kipper' necktie, 1977.

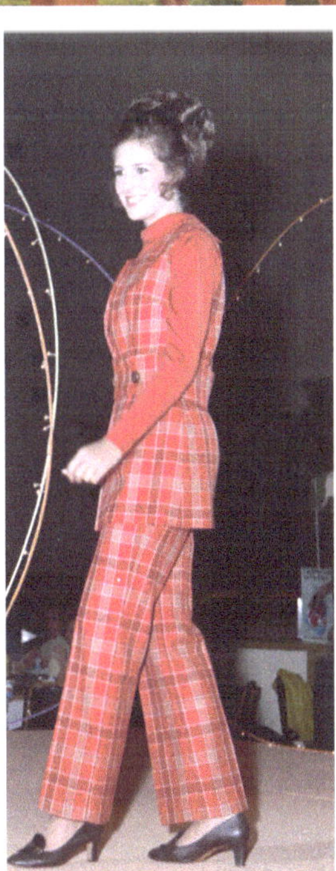

Above: mini-dresses, 1971.

Left: plaid pants suit, 1970.

Fashion in the 1970s (continued)

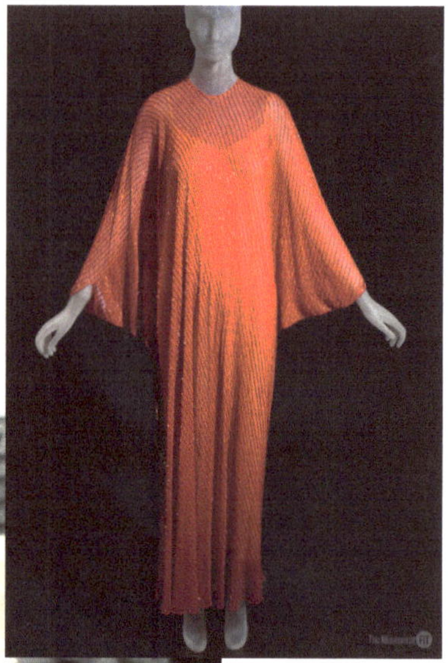

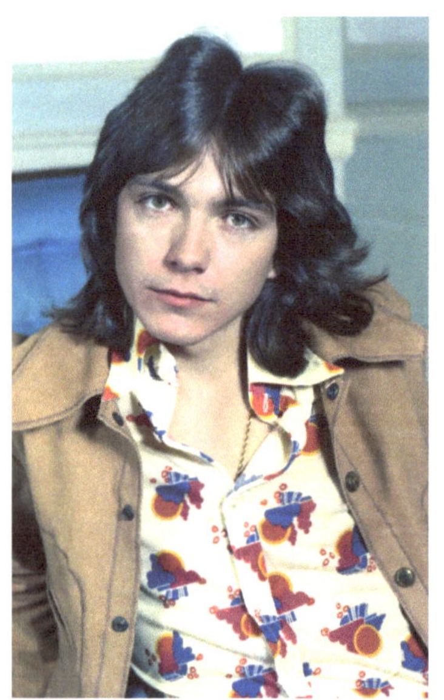

Above: singer David Cassidy with typical 70s hairstyle and shirt.

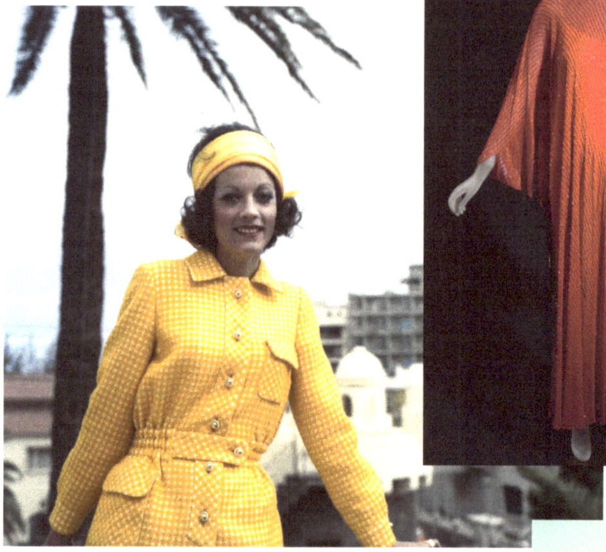

Right: kaftan, 1976.

Above: coat dress with matching bandana, 1973.

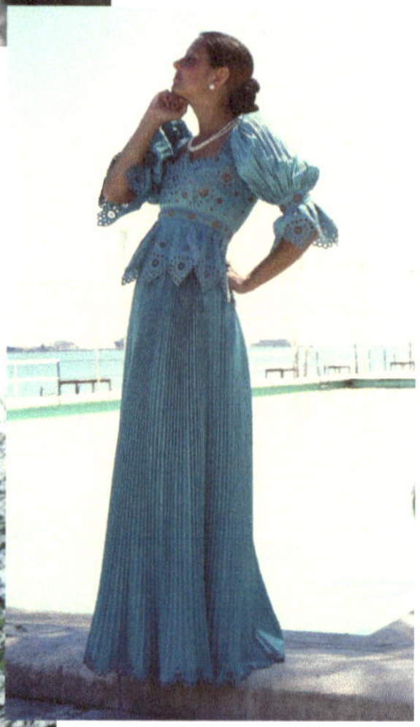

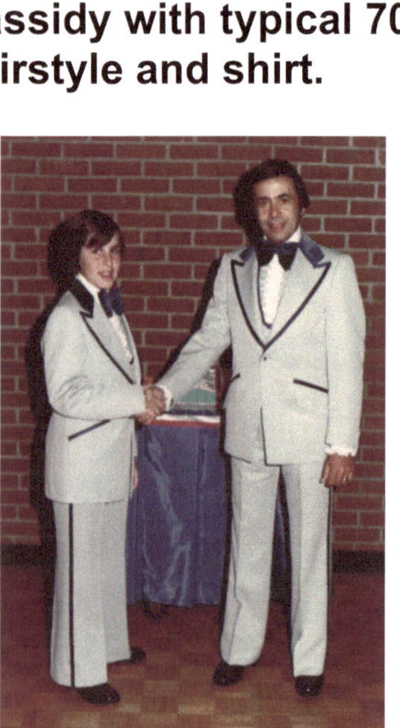

Above: father and son in powder blue tuxedos, 1976.

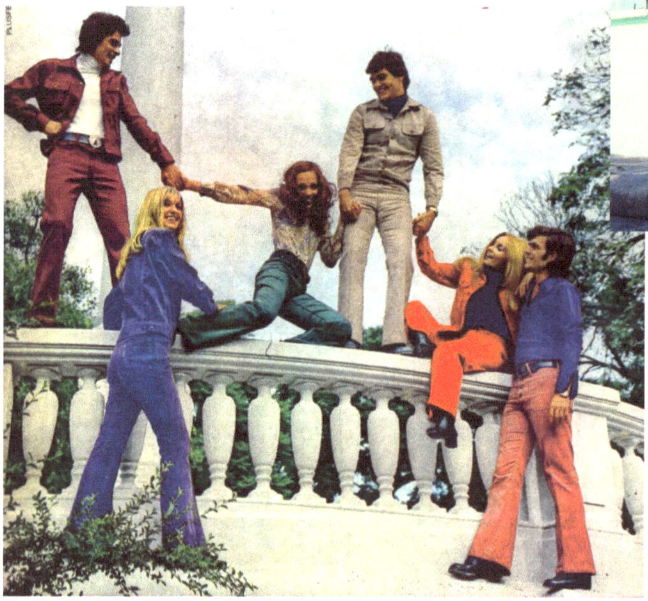

Above: unisex styles, 1972.

Above: Victorian style maxi dress, 1973.

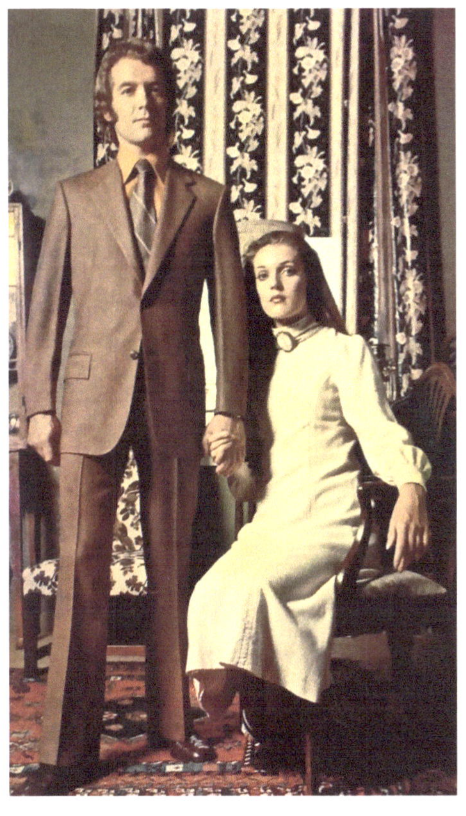

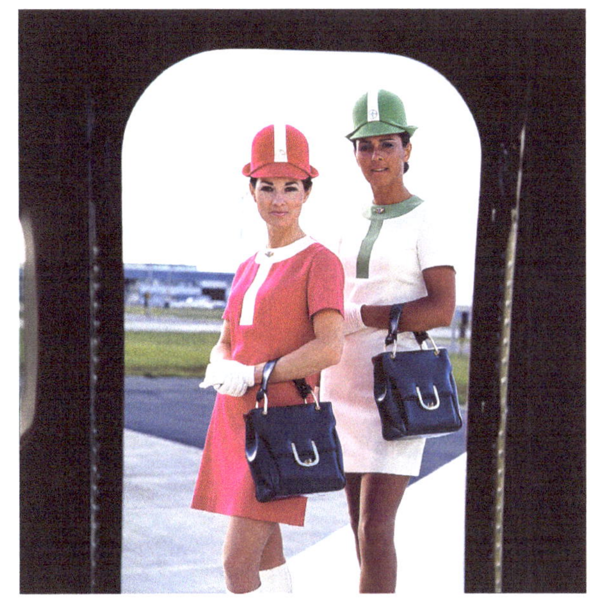

Left:
Air
hostesses,
1970.

Left: Man in polyester suit with
woman in maxi dress, 1973.

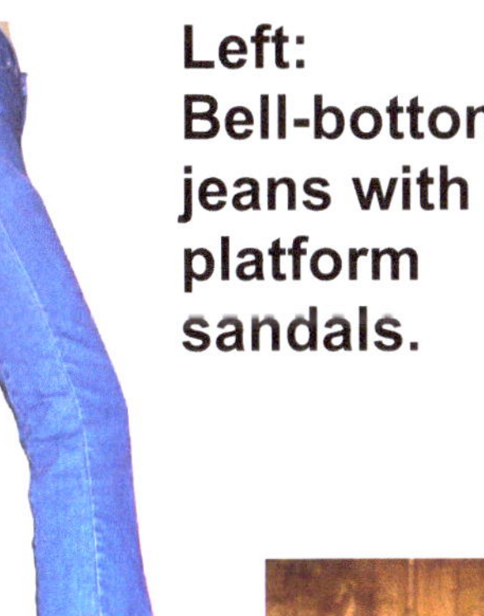

Left:
Bell-bottom
jeans with
platform
sandals.

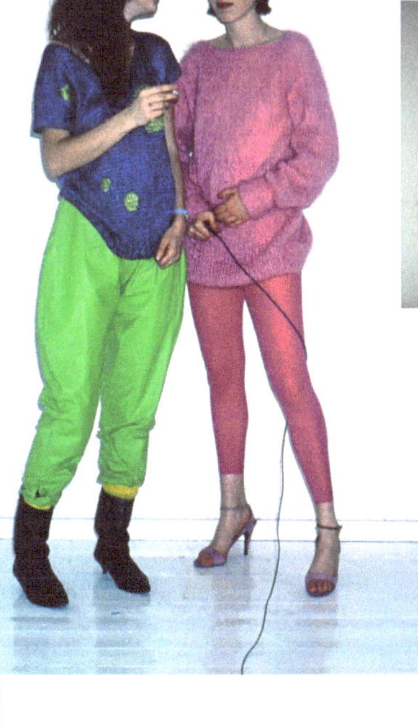

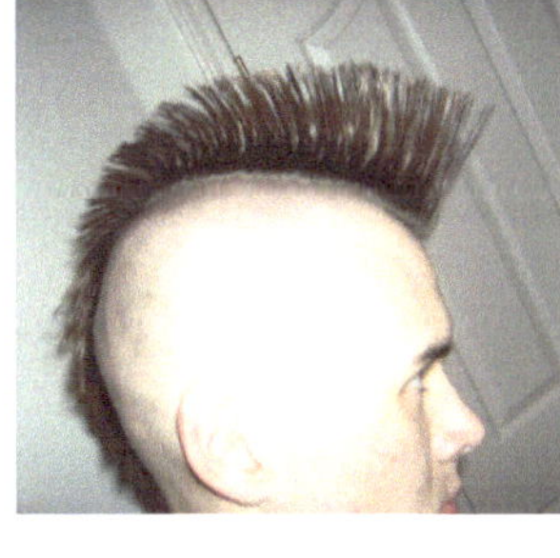

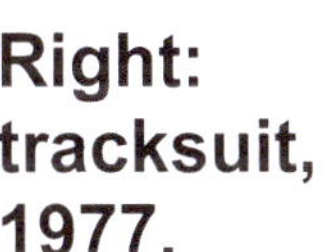

Right:
tracksuit,
1977.

Above: disco wear, 1979.
Above right: man with 'mohawk'
hairstyle, late 1970s.

Technology in the 1970s

The growth in consumer technology which started in the 1950s continued into the 1970s as household gadgets and consumer durables got bigger, better and cheaper.

An important area of technological change was home entertainment; color TV, home video recorders, video games and cassette tape players all became widely available during the decade.

Kitchen and laundry technology also improved and many new gadgets were found in homes, such as microwave ovens, electric can openers, tumble dryers and electric sewing machines

Home improvements were popular in the 1970s and this led to increased sales of power tools such as drills and saws. The first calculators and home computers also appeared in the 1970s.

Above: Singer sewing machine.

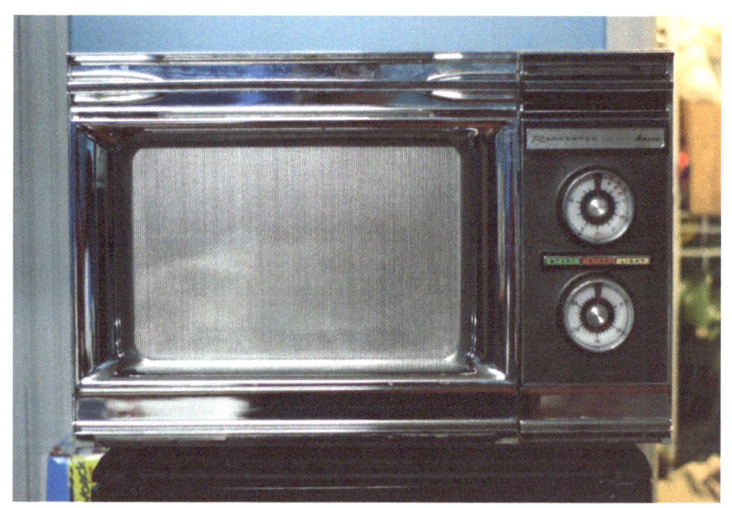

Above: Electronic (microwave) oven, 1974.

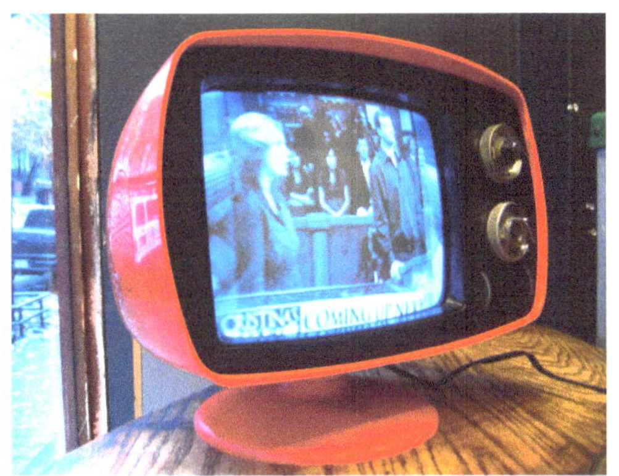

Above: portable TV set.
Below: TV game console.

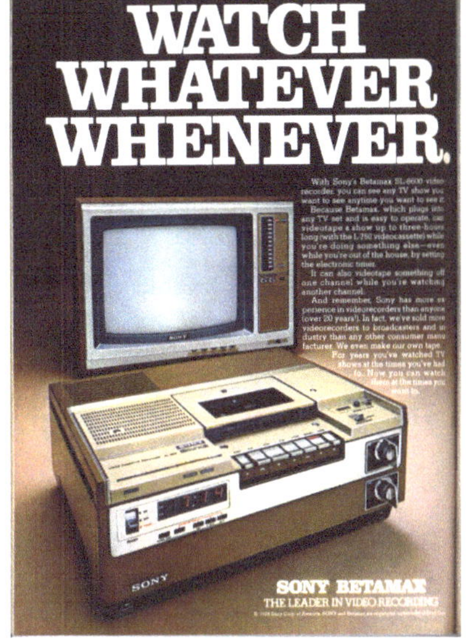

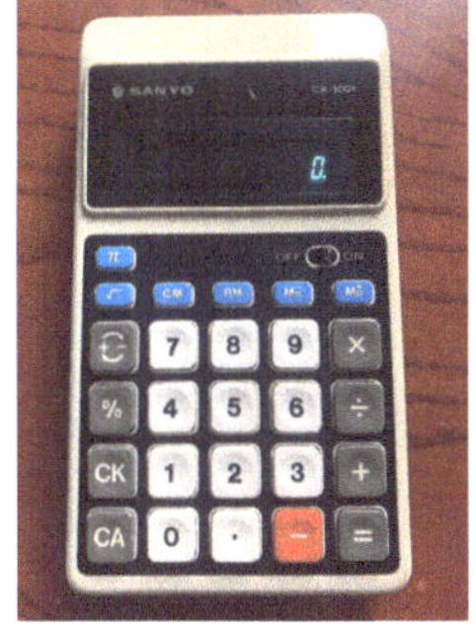

Above: pocket calculator.

Left: Home video recorder (VCR).

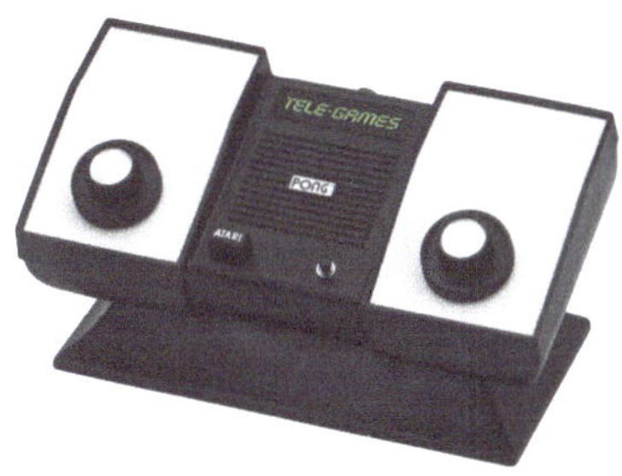

Right: portable record player with auto-changer turntable

Below: AT&T push button phone.

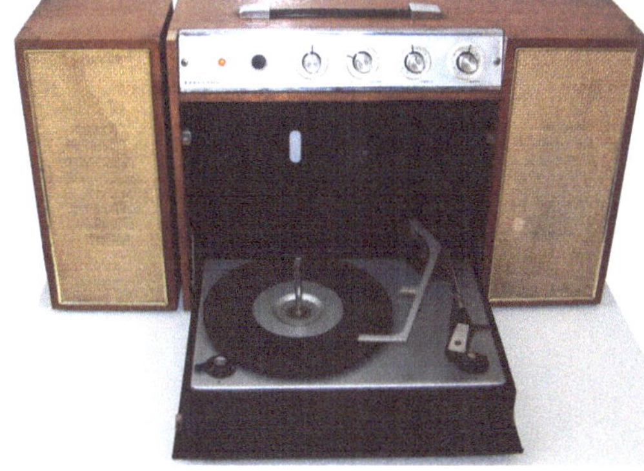

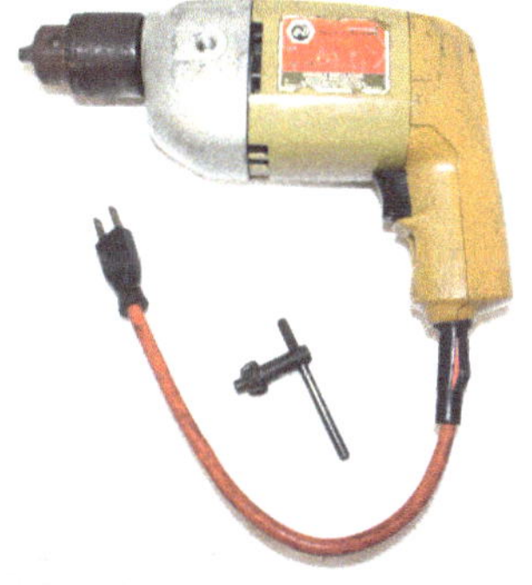

Above: Black and Decker electric drill.

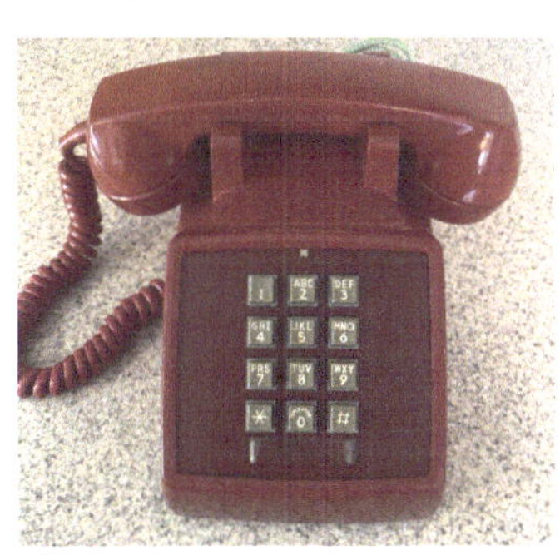

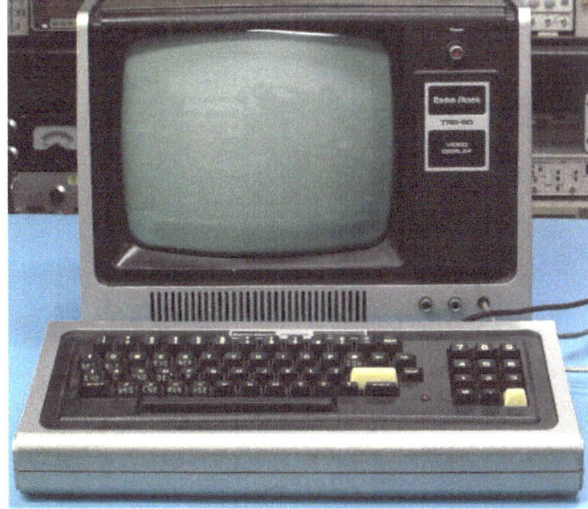

Above: Radio Shack TRS-80 home computer (1977).

Left: cassette player with cassette tape.

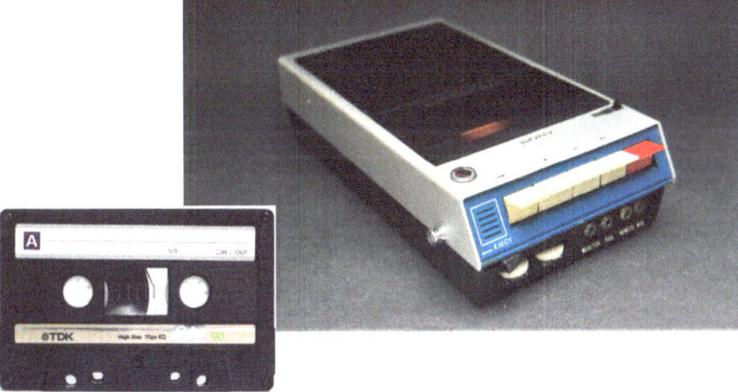

People in the 1970s

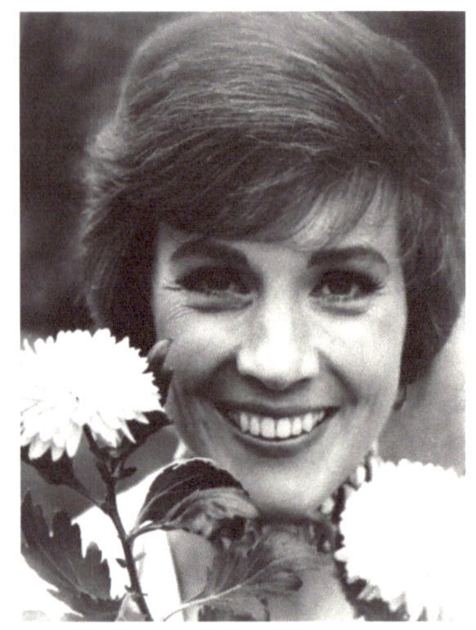

Actress Julie Andrews, 1970.

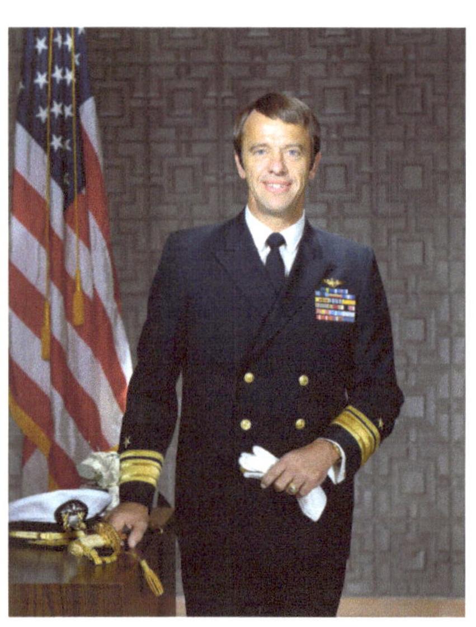

Astronaut Alan Shephard, 1971.

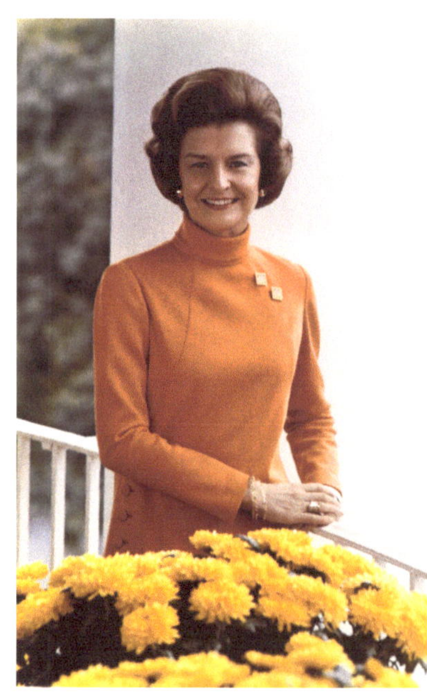

Betty Ford, First Lady, 1974.

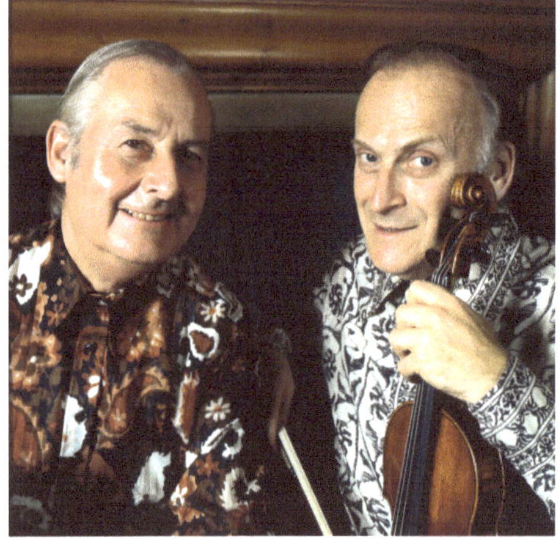

Musicians Yehudi Menuhin and Stephane Grapelli, 1976.

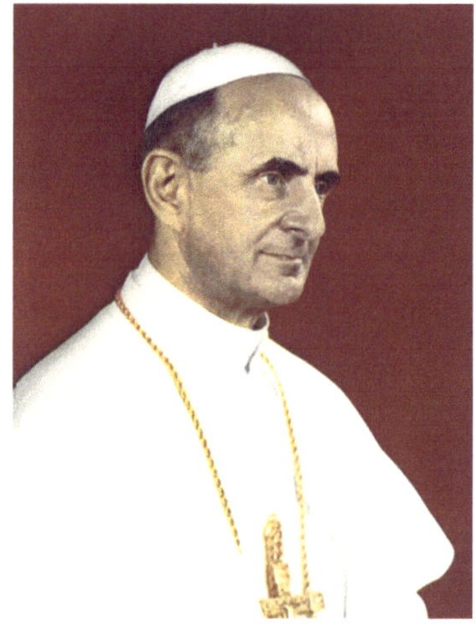

Pope Paul VI, (1963-1978).

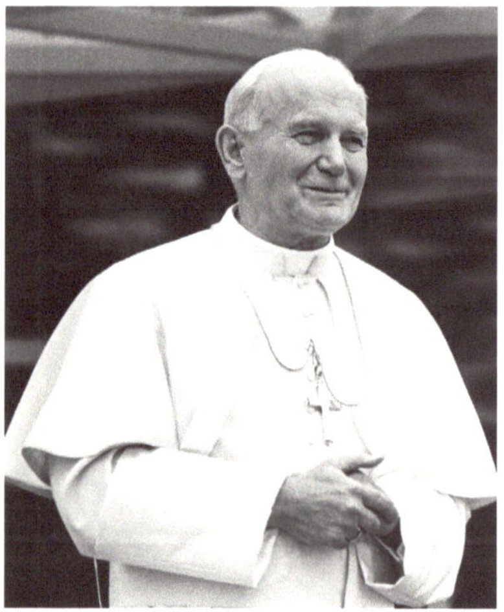

Pope John Paul II, (1978-2005).

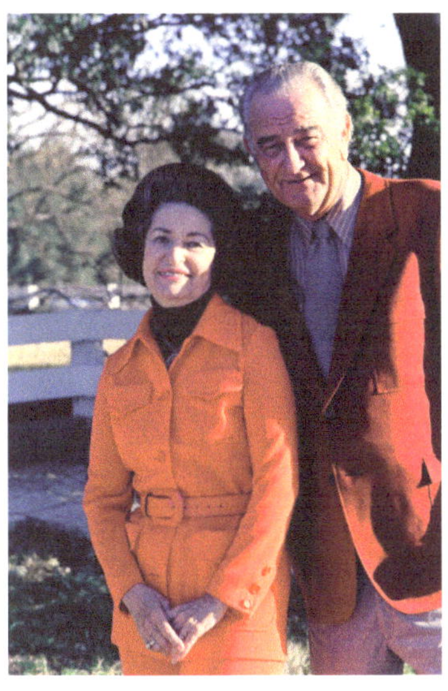

Former President Lydon B Johnson with his wife 'Lady Bird', 1972.

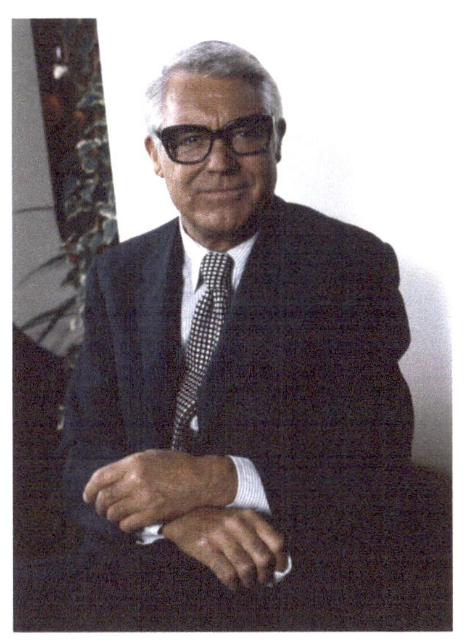

Actor Cary Grant, 1973.

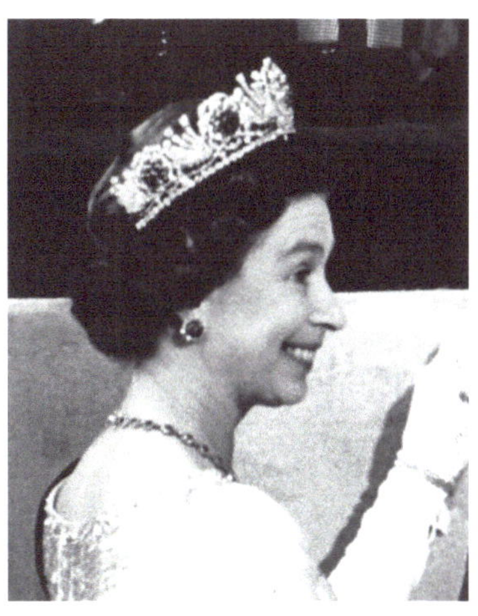

Queen Elizabeth II, 1977.

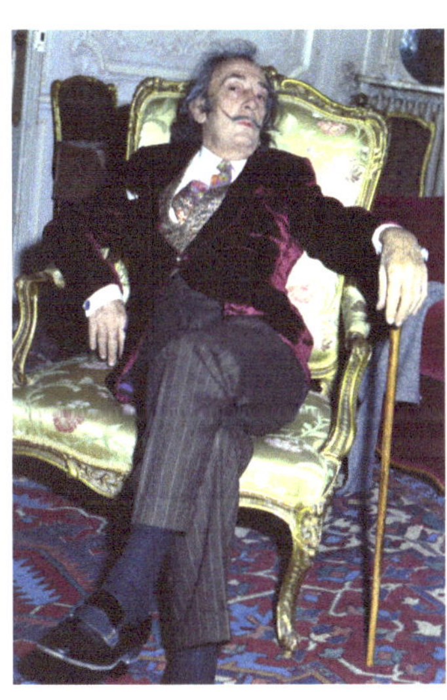

Artist Salvador Dali, 1972.

Right: Singer Bing Crosby, 1977.

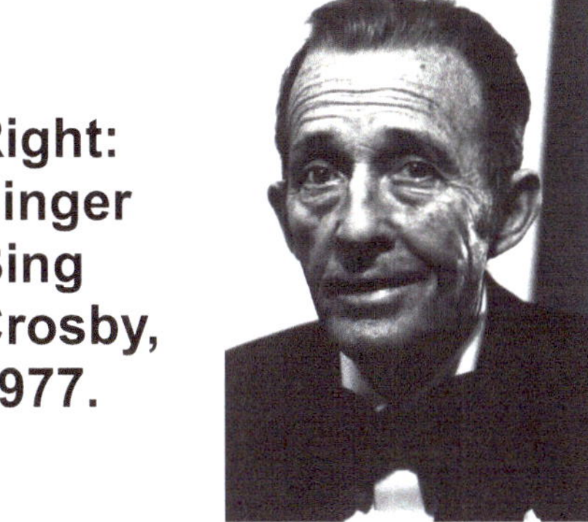

Below: President Nixon and First Lady Pat Nixon meet with California Governor Ronald Reagan and his wife Nancy, 1970.

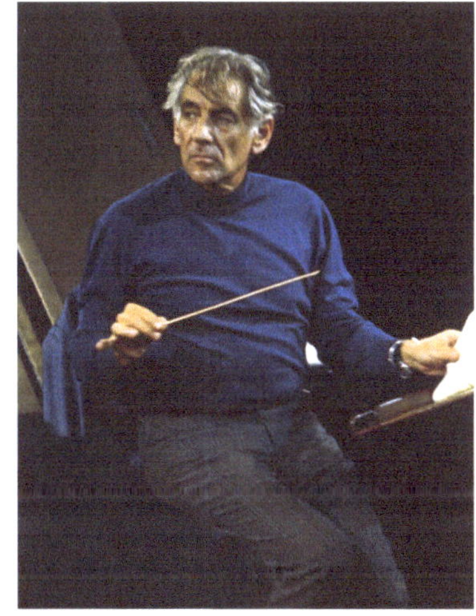

Conductor Leonard Bernstein, 1973.

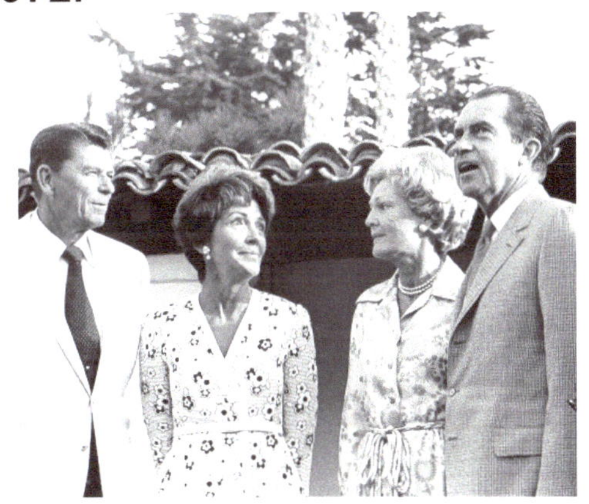

The Shah of Iran and Queen Farah, 1977.

Events of the 1970s

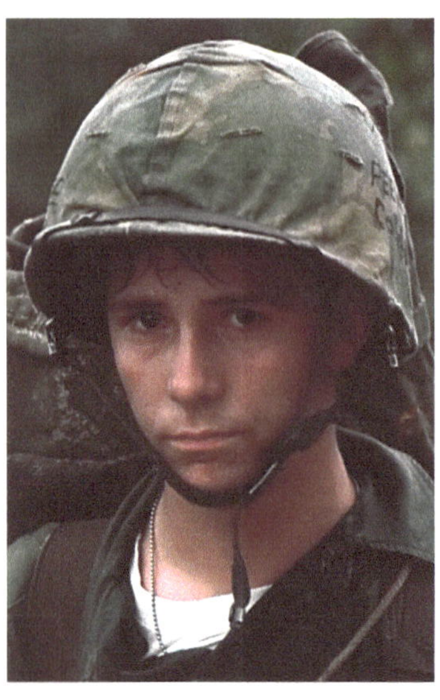

Left: a US Marine in Vietnam. The US military pulled out of the war in 1973.

Below: anti-war protesters led by veterans.

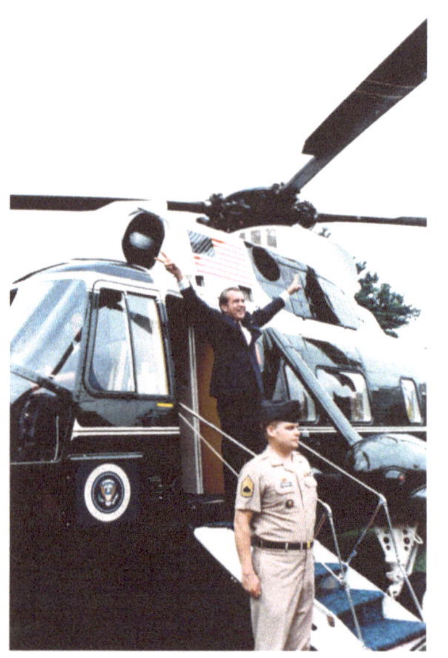

Above: President Nixon leaves the White House in 1974 after resigning in the wake of the Watergate scandal.

Below: astronaut Eugene Cernan drives the Lunar Rover on the last manned mission to the moon in 1972.

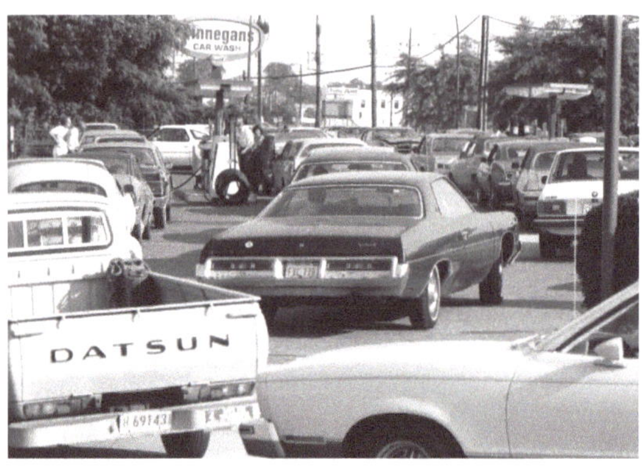

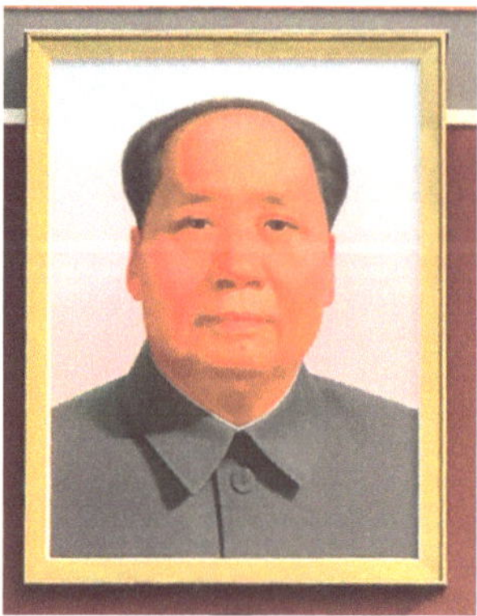

Below: Chinese leader Chairman Mao.

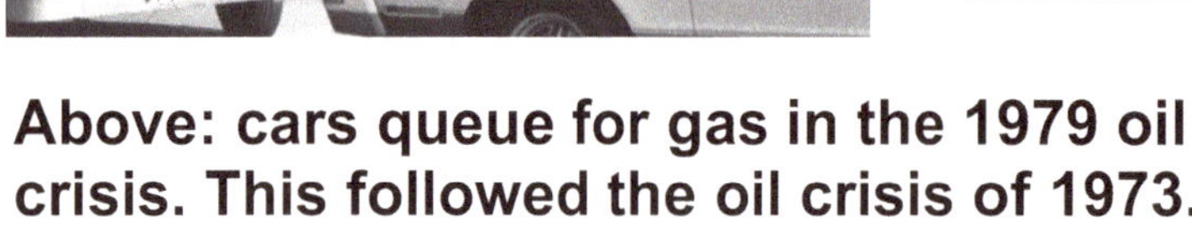

Above: cars queue for gas in the 1979 oil crisis. This followed the oil crisis of 1973.

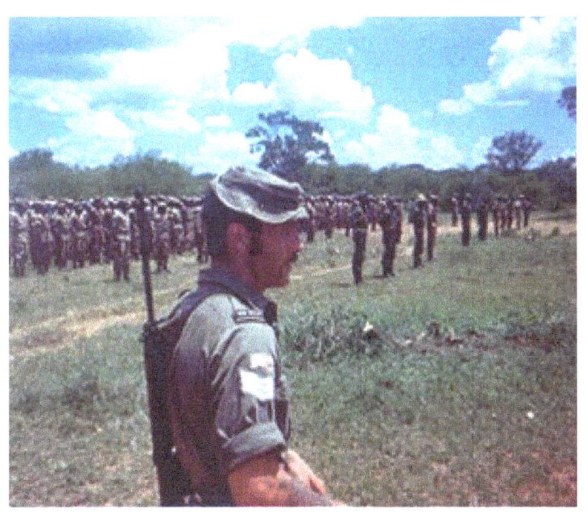

Left: a soldier during the 1964-1979 civil war in the former British colony of Rhodesia.

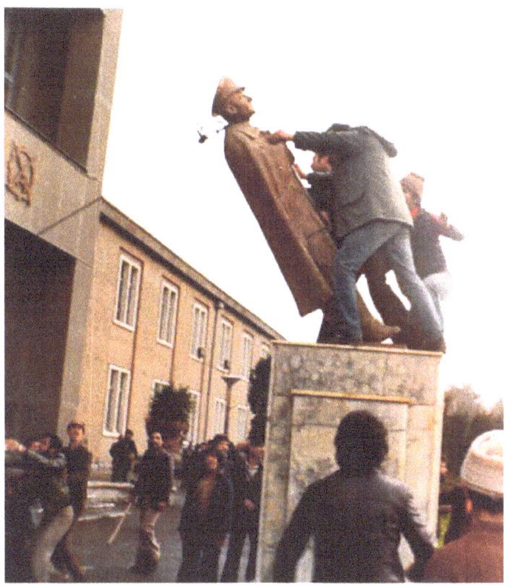

Above: a statue of the Shah of Persia is torn down during the 1979 Iranian revolution.

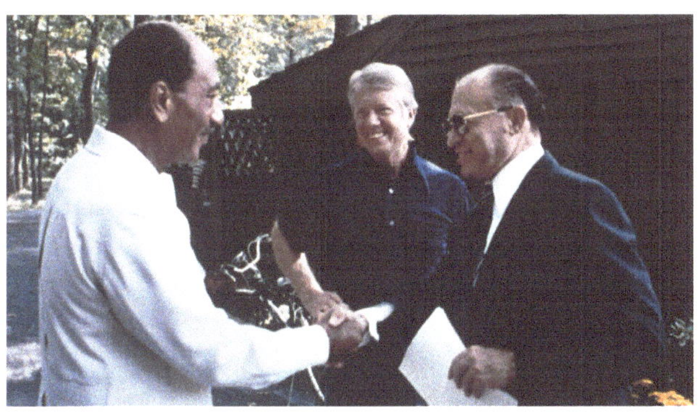

Above: Egypt's Anwar Sadat and Israel's Menacham Begin with President Carter agree to the Camp David peace treaty in 1978 .

Right: NASA's first space station, Skylab, went into orbit in 1973.

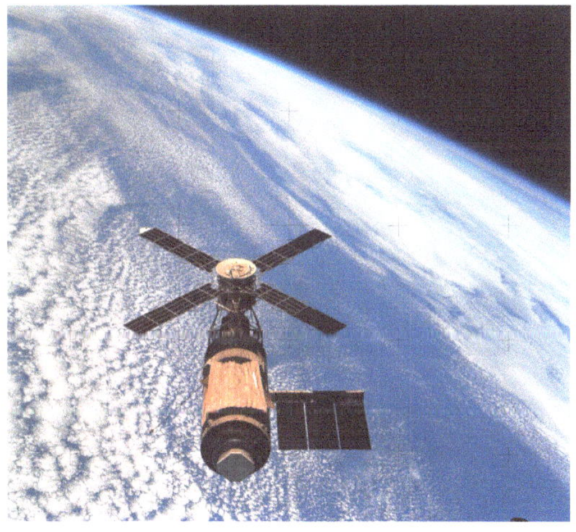

Below: Margaret Thatcher became Britain's first woman prime minister in 1979.

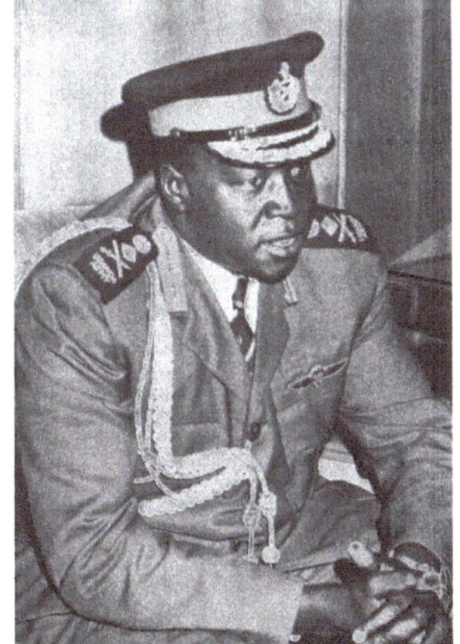

Above: the dictator Idi Amin seized power in Uganda in 1971.

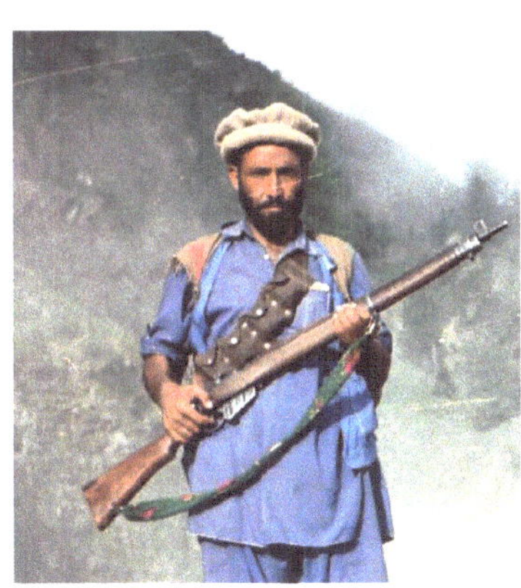

Above: an Afghan tribesman. The USSR invaded Afghanistan in 1979.

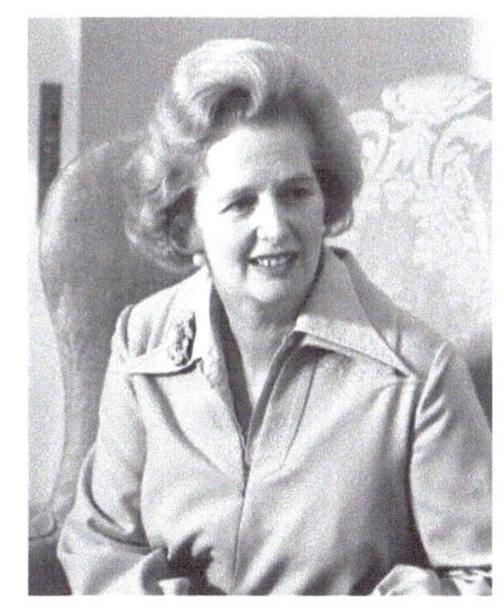

Other **Memory Lane** titles

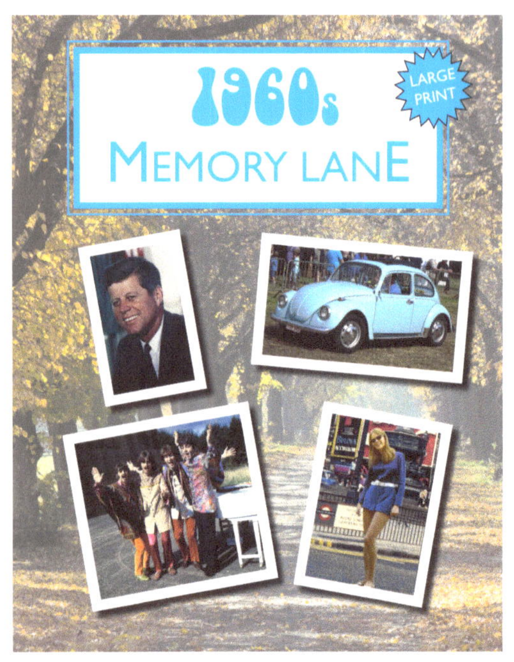

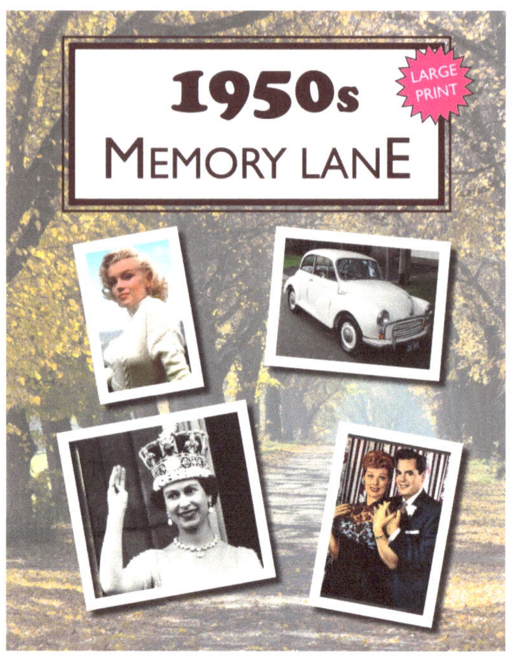

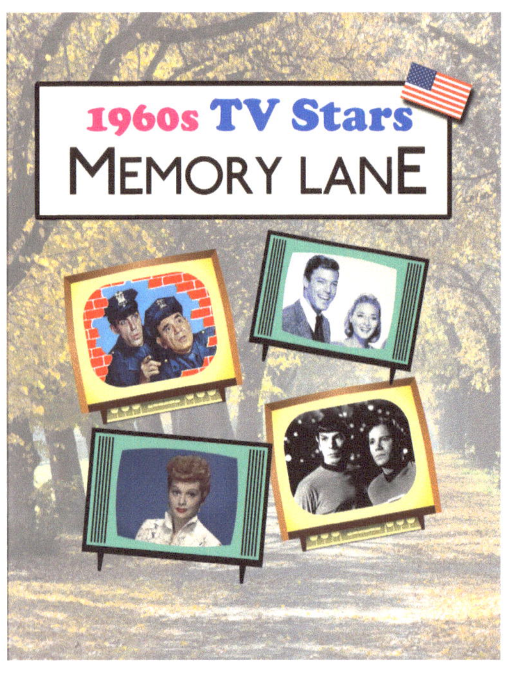

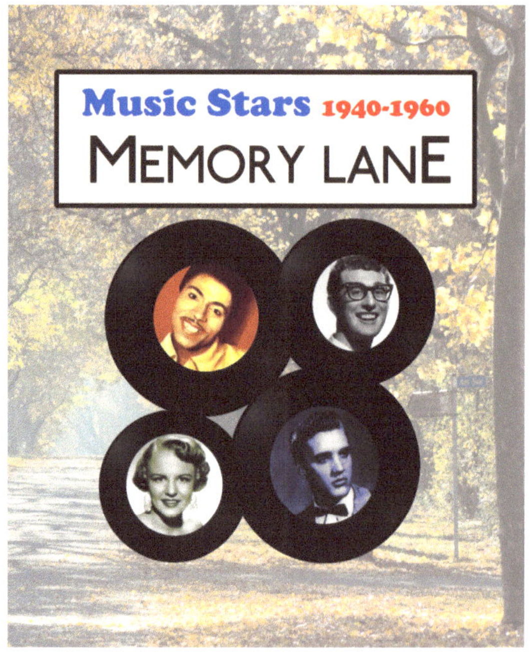

Available at Amazon.com

or order from your local bookstore